ALONE

DANIEL SCHREIBER

Translation by Ben Fergusson

REAKTION BOOKS

Published by
REAKTION BOOKS LTD
Unit 32, Waterside
44–48 Wharf Road
London N1 7UX, UK
www.reaktionbooks.co.uk

First published 2023
Copyright © Daniel Schreiber 2023
Translation from the German by Ben Fergusson 2022
Allein by Daniel Schreiber
© 2021 Hanser Berlin in der Carl Hanser Verlag GmbH & Co. KG, Munich

The translation of this work was supported by a grant from the Goethe-Institut

Printed and bound in Great Britain by TJ Books Ltd, Padstow, Cornwall

A catalogue record for this book is available from the British Library

ISBN 978 1 78914 765 0

The quote on p. 7 is from *The Years* by Annie Ernaux. Translated from the
French by Alison L. Strayer © Editions Gallimard, Paris, 2008 © the English
edition Fitzcarraldo Editions, London, 7th edition, 2021, p. 97.

Contents

At every moment in time, next to the things it seems natural to do and say . . . are the other things that society hushes up without knowing it is doing so. Thus it condemns to lonely suffering all the people who feel but cannot name these things. Then the silence breaks, little by little, or suddenly one day, and the words burst forth, recognised at last, while underneath other silences start to form.

ANNIE ERNAUX, *The Years*

Living Alone

We sat around the back of the house on rickety folding chairs, drank coffee, enjoyed the last warm rays of the late summer sun and looked out over the overgrown plot that had once been a large allotment. Sylvia and Heiko had built the house near a lake, Liepnitzsee, in the countryside outside of Berlin. It had taken a few years to complete everything, but they had now moved in with their little daughter Lilith and had finally turned their backs on their lives in Berlin. I had mixed feelings about their move. I wasn't sure what this new physical distance would mean for my social life and, in particular, for my long-standing friendship with Sylvia.

No one had taken care of the garden in years. In front of us lay a dishevelled field of dry grasses, milkweed and stinging nettles, surrounded by huge, densely packed thuja conifers. In the middle of the garden, three great pines towered up into the sky, with a few scrawny cherry laurels and rhododendron bushes peppered in between, their branches bulky, their leaves sparse. The only plants able to hold their own were a few surprisingly drought-resistant purple rose campions, some pink cranesbill and bright amber heliopsis. On the spur of the moment, I asked Sylvia if she wanted me to help her redesign the garden. I couldn't say exactly why this felt right in that moment. It was something to do with the hope that working in nature, with plants, might help ground me. Perhaps a part of me saw my own life mirrored in the disastrous state of that garden: disastrous despite the many touches of beauty. In the months leading up to that moment, I had increasingly been feeling as if something had gone wrong; as if, in my youth, I had succumbed to some kind of dreamy misconception about adult life. And that the effects of this misconception were only just becoming apparent.

I NEVER MADE A conscious decision to live alone. On the contrary, for the longest time I had assumed that I would share my life with someone and that we would grow old together. I have always been in relationships – shorter, longer, very long; relationships that often merged into one another. I lived with two of my partners and, with one of them, spent years planning a future together. During that phase of my life, the weeks in which I was single often felt like an eternity; an eternity that I filled with affairs and one-night stands, with romantic obsessions that I only think back with reluctance. But at some point in time it all ended. Months passed, then years, in which I wasn't in a relationship, in which I had fewer and fewer affairs. Having been unable to be alone, I suddenly found myself seeking out solitude.

When I talked to my friends about this change, I explained to them that, when I was younger, I was more open-minded and more willing to take risks. Sometimes I would say that the world of gay love and desire was characterized by a mercilessness that, after a certain age, made you invisible. But I also wondered whether I was simply too psychologically overburdened to have another relationship, whether I even had room for it in my life. A life in which I had to work so hard just to keep my head above water and in which I needed so much time for my real passion: writing.

This was all true, of course, but as an explanation it fell short. Because on some days I also thought that I was by myself because I lacked a kind of fundamental optimism. Ultimately, I didn't feel as if I had a good or promising future ahead of me, a future worth sharing. This helplessness was by no means limited to my private life. The consequences of insurmountable economic inequality, the growing influence of autocratic regimes, climate change that was almost certainly irreversible – I felt that humanity had lost the will to confront the catastrophes it was facing. Instead, we seemed to be surrendering to them with an oddly cheerful fatalism. Every drought-filled summer, every tropical storm that destroyed whole swathes of land and whole island states, every forecast of another refugee crisis stoked by famine and the subsequent political collapse, every news item about the inaction of the world's governments made me feel even more hopeless. Whenever I read about the surprising successes of political disinformation campaigns, the warnings of cyberattacks and bioterrorism, of new viruses and global epidemics about to catch us unawares, this feeling of hopelessness intensified.

Perhaps what I felt could best be best described as a 'moral injury'. The term comes from studies on war reporters suffering from post-traumatic stress disorder and describes a violation of one's inner understanding of reality. It occurs when one has to witness horrific events but one is unable to intervene.[1] Although most of our lives are, of course, not comparable to the lives of those who report from the front line, they are shaped by a similar dilemma. We follow the horrors of what is happening in our world and we are largely condemned to inaction. For a long time now, it has seemed to me to be almost impossible not to experience this as a painful attack on my moral compass, on my understanding of myself and the world.

I LOVE GARDENS. Even as a small child, I asked my mother – a passionate gardener – to tell me the names of plants and I would lose myself for hours playing among the huge fruit trees and feathery asparagus. I have been regularly going to Bornim near Potsdam to see the beautiful historic garden of Karl Foerster, the legendary nursery-man who bred perennial plants. In Versailles, I can walk for hours through Jean-Baptiste de la Quintinies Potager du roi. I am always blown away by Sissinghurst Castle, the country estate and sprawling gardens of Vita Sackville-West, in which plants are arranged by the colour of their flowers. In recent years, I have been particularly fascinated by the work of the Dutch garden designer Piet Oudolf. His gardens are wildly beautiful. They resemble rhythmic seas of prairie plants, native perennials and grasses, in which something is always in bloom and which, due to the distinctive shapes of some of the plants, are inviting even in winter.

Oudolf's gardens spoke to me in a way that was difficult to put into words. They not only satisfied my need for sanctuary, they also gave me the feeling that something could be done about the adver-sities we face in the world today. They revealed to me a way to make the world, at least within the confines of a single plot of land, a little more beautiful and to lay in a small way the foundations for a better future. They seemed to reveal a possibility of living with and in a world that we struggle with.

INSPIRED BY OUDOLF and his gardening philosophy, I suggested to Sylvia and Heiko that we redesign their garden around their house on a much grander scale. I got my hands on all of Oudolf's books and worked through them methodically. The goal was to create an ecologically sustainable garden that, year on year, would require less work because the plants were so well matched that they would form a kind of mini ecosystem. A garden that only needed a minimum of watering, even during hot summers.

Little by little, we set to work. I had a key to the house. Whenever I needed to travel up, or even just when I wasn't feeling great, I would get on the local train and go up to Liepnitzsee. When I was there, I would get up early, make myself a coffee and go outside. Working with my hands also entailed a kind of psychological work; the tilling of the space of the garden was accompanied by an expansion of my mental space. Or at least that's what it felt like to me.[2]

THAT AUTUMN, I often found myself thinking about Jean-François Lyotard's famous thesis on the 'end of grand narratives'. It was a notion that Lyotard had put forward in the late 1970s in his book *The Postmodern Condition*. Lyotard's 'grand narratives' were not literary narratives; instead, he was describing the ways in which our society had suffered from a fundamental loss of credibility. The 'narratives' that he had in mind were those of politics and philosophy. In his opinion, these fields could no longer lay claim to any kind of authoritative 'rationale'.[3]

I had the impression that we were only just beginning to experience, in real life, what the end of these great narratives actually meant; that we had, in fact, been able to follow it in real time for some years now. It was reflected in developments that were sometimes welcome, sometimes deeply threatening. The end of unchallenged patriarchy and rigid notions of gender, for instance. But also the apparent end of collective responsibility, of social action underpinned by science, of a shared belief in democracy.

For Lyotard, the collapse of our grand narratives also called into question the 'autonomous subject' able to rely on self-evident certainties and to say what is right and what is wrong based on universally shared truths. Instead, he saw the emergence of an individuals who were left to cope alone, who had to navigate their own way through a multiplicity of 'little narratives'. They became searching selves who confronted the fundamental changes of our age by living a life of lost certainties, craving new beliefs. This idea of the searching self was something I could completely identify with.

Perhaps the last grand narrative to have survived these shifts is that of romantic love. Or at least its rudiments. It is true that we are slowly leaving behind the 'divine' and 'natural' order of the sexes that, for a long time, were part of this grand narrative. It is of course also true that what we conceive of as 'love' has fundamentally changed. Sociologists like Eva Illouz have written compellingly about how our notion of love is affected by the commercialization of our feelings, the capitalization of our bodies, the whole emotional attention economy – always searching for something more, something better.[4] And yet, the idea of love has lost hardly any of its allure. It continues to be the focus of our collective fantasies. Its place in our personal horizons remains fixed. It is still what most people desire and what they hope for. It is, perhaps, the most essential component of what they understand happiness to be. For most of us, a life without the intimacy of love is incomplete, unfulfilled – a life that is fundamentally missing something.

These days, our unhappiness is often understood as a result of individual failure, despite the fact that unhappiness can represent a completely appropriate reaction to the world and the society we live in. The lack of a romantic relationship is generally seen as a kind of personal failure in the same vein, as the consequence of a lack of attractiveness, a lack of professional success, a lack of physical fitness. When you live alone, you are constantly stumbling into these free-floating assumptions, not least in the faces of other people, in their pity, their projections of shame, sometimes even in their secret joy that they are better off than you.

PERHAPS THIS PERCEPTION is one of the reasons why we still know so little about the everyday lives and mental health of people who live alone. As the psychotherapist Julia Samuel points out in her book *This Too Shall Pass*, up until now the focus of psychological research has always been on romantic partnerships, on the lives of people living in a couple. Remarkably, there is barely any research on how people cope with living alone.[5] After all, now more than ever, we are encouraged to put ourselves in the centre of our own life plan. 'Individual autonomy' and 'self-realization' have become collective ideals.[6] The great array of different ways of living has become so much wider; traditional family ties have loosened. Marriages and conventional romantic relationships have become shorter and more unstable than they once were. More people live alone now, in fact, than at any other time in history.[7] People like me. Many of us have not found a partner, have not started a family, even if those were things that we once desired. Many of us, willingly or not, have said goodbye to the grand narrative of love – even if some of us still believe in it.

Whether we are in a relationship or not, we all still have a need for a sense of intimacy that has to be fulfilled. Without being able to put it into words, I felt, when I was with Sylvia and her family at Liepnitzsee, that I was not as caught up with myself and my life alone as I normally was. Contrary to my fears when they first moved, we were in fact spending a lot of time together. At the weekends, when we devoted ourselves to the big jobs in the garden, we would sit around a fire, pleasantly exhausted, or would retreat to their large kitchen, cook, eat, try to convince Lilith to eat the odd vegetable, play cards with her. To calm the waves surging within, it helps to spend time in the company of people one knows well and whom one trusts.[8]

In a sense, our work together in Sylvia's garden represented a new chapter in our friendship; the continuation of a long story that we are both still writing, a story with highs and lows, intensive phases and new beginnings. I have known Sylvia since I was twelve. We prepped for our physics and history exams together, headed out to the lakes or went out together in town. She was the first person I told that I was gay. When we were nineteen we travelled through Italy for six weeks with camping equipment strapped to our backs, smoked joints on the beaches of Calabria, had laughing fits and both flirted with the same cellist – a man who gave us a private concert in his parents' house, surrounded by orange and lemon trees. We lived together in our first flat in Berlin. After I moved to New York, I would stay with her in Kreuzberg when I was visiting Germany. A few days after Lilith was born, I held her in my arms and, later, became her godfather.

Sylvia is one of the few people who not only knows who I am, but also knows who I was ten or twenty years ago. We change, we change all the time. And we forget, forget even when we don't want to, who we once were. We need people around us to remind us, to keep us from forgetting.

WHEN YOU LIVE ALONE, it is friendships, like the one I share with Sylvia, that often form the centre of your life. The relationships that I have with many of my friends have lasted longer than my longest romantic relationships. These friendships are the source of my greatest conflicts as well as my greatest joys. Some of my friendships are based on common interests, on shared season tickets to the Berlin Philharmonic or the Berlin State Opera, on exchanging reading and exhibition tips. I've been friends with some of these people for so long that, when we're asked how long we've known each other, we just laugh in embarrassment. Other friendships are more recent. My oldest friend is over seventy, my youngest in her mid-twenties. It is friendships that structure my life. It is friends with whom I share it.

So much is written about the grand narrative of romantic love, so many films are made about it and so many theories are developed to explain it that we often disregard other narratives of closeness and intimacy, or do not afford them the importance they deserve. Even if we don't form long-term romantic relationships, even if we don't have kids, even if we go through life alone: we almost always have friendships. And for many of us, as the philosopher Marilyn Friedman points out, they are among the most uncontested, enduring and satisfying of all of our close, personal bonds.[9]

Friendships are the only relationships we have that are entirely voluntary, based on two people mutually agreeing to share ideas, spend time with each other and be there for each other, to varying degrees. Unlike family relationships, with their rituals and obligations, you are not born into friendships. And they are rarely based on the same kinds of rules of exclusivity that govern romantic relationships, nor are they beholden to the same agendas of desire. We choose our friends based on who they are, and we, in turn, are chosen on the exact same basis.

NOWADAYS, friendships often have a different urgency than romantic relationships. It is something that the sociologist Sasha Roseneil has uncovered in her research. Modern friendships, she writes, are part of our 'practices of self-repair'. They can help us 'heal the wounds of the self' and confront 'mental distress, disappointment, psychological suffering and loss'. They can ensure that our lives are not completely dominated by emotional distress or the fallout of failed relationships.[10]

Yet, what we talk about when we talk about friendship is different for each and every one of us. In fact, when it comes to those relationships that we describe as friendships, it is striking how diverse the forms they can take are.[11] According to the most recent sociological research, friendships should not, in fact, be understood as a single type of relationship, but rather as a 'family of abstract forms of relationships', a 'gradiated web of related social forms'.[12] These can range from short-lived acquaintances to long-term, intimate relationships. There are people with large circles of friends and those with small ones. While some people fill their lives with intense friendships, making a clear distinction between 'real friends' and 'acquaintances', others have many different types of friends and try to 'balance' their relationships according to their needs. Some people rely on their friends for the long haul; others change their circle of friends at each new stage of their lives.[13] The secret of friendships lies in their great diversity, in the fact that they are able to encompass so much more than any one of us can imagine.

Perhaps it is our difficulty in clearly defining friendships that causes us to attach less importance to them than to family relationships and romantic relationships. Only love is able to claim a grand narrative for itself. Friendships revolve around small narratives, countless small narratives unwilling to follow preordained patterns or contractual characteristics.

I NEVER DREAMT of being alone. I never dreamt that friendships, rather than a relationship and a family, would be the most important spheres of intimacy for me. But I still like my life; I like the many people I am close to; I like my flat, my balcony overflowing with plants; I like the time I have to travel, to cook for people, to wander around town sometimes for hours on end. I like that there is room in my life for projects like the garden at Liepnitzsee. Even without a romantic relationship, my life often feels fulfilled. And yet, despite everything, there remains a void, a trace of longing. Every now and again, briefly, I wish I had a partner, someone to spend a relaxing weekend with, someone to wake up next to me in the morning, who asks me in the evening how my day was, someone I can tell what time I'll be home, someone who holds me when I'm sad. I wonder whether I'm missing something fundamental but can't admit it to myself. Whether I have become so good at living alone that I no longer notice my loneliness. Whether the fragile balance of my life is grounded in me unwittingly repressing my longing, repressing my desire.

Reflecting on Joan Didion's famous phrase, 'We tell ourselves stories in order to live', essayist Maggie Nelson writes that it is stories that 'may enable us to live, but they also trap us'. 'In their scramble to make sense of nonsensical things,' Nelson writes, 'they distort, codify, blame, aggrandise, restrict, omit, betray, mythologise, you name it.'[14] I'm not sure how right she is. But I do believe that we have to keep returning to the stories we tell ourselves to make sure that they still ; that we sometimes have to discard them in order to be able to retell them afresh or find new stories that do fit.

The reason that all of these explanations for my solitude felt wrong was the pervasive assumption of my own passivity. Again and again, I framed it as something that had 'happened' to me. But couldn't it also be the case that I had sought out this life alone? Or at least a part of me had, a part that I didn't want to acknowledge? The part of me that was afraid of the hurt that would inevitably come with a relationship, that wanted to avoid the long depressions that would follow a potential break up, that couldn't stand the necessary compromises, the frictions of everyday life. The part, then, that didn't let many people get close to it. Maybe I lived alone because I wanted to live alone.

But can you really live a good life alone, without a romantic relationship? Can our need for intimacy be satisfied by friendships? How sustainable is a model like that? And how does one deal with those moments in which, at some point, most of one's friends have found partners and one finds oneself even alone in living alone? In other words, how do you learn to live with being alone without it hurting, without lying to yourself? These were the questions that I didn't know the answers to.

WE CONTINUED TO GARDEN until the onset of winter. We cut down the thuja conifers, cleared large parts of the plot, created a lawn and flower bed, raised beds for vegetables and areas for fruit trees. We cultivated the soil, planted fragrant hawthorn, lilac bushes, weigelas, snowy Mespilus, red-leaved elder, black cherry plum trees and old-fashioned mock orange along the perimeter. We put countless bulbs in the ground – wild tulips, old pheasant's eye, striped squills, snowdrops, crocuses and winter aconites – and planted hellebores and Lenten roses, largeleaf Brunneras, grasses, ferns, wild fennel, profuse perovskias, shade-loving astilbes and many other hardy perennials.

The effort felt good. People, says cultural historian Robert Harrison in his book *Gardens*, were not created to ponder the turmoil, the death and the endless suffering of their history. They create gardens to find refuge from the tumult of the ages. It is, in fact, Harrison argues, precisely because we are thrown into this history that we have to cultivate our own garden. So that we can discover the healing power within us, so that we can preserve our humanity.[15] When you cultivate a garden, the future is uncertain. You don't know what your plot will look like in a few months', years' or decades' time, whether what you plant and sow will eventually flourish and bloom. You lay the foundations for something, you water, you fertilize, you weed, you learn to live with setbacks and to let go. Gardening is not only an expression of hope; it is also a very concrete act of hope.

PERHAPS THESE ARE ultimately the reasons why we cultivate friendships too, especially in a life lived alone: so as not to lose our grip on reality, to counter the passage of time and rampant entropy, in order to create the possibility of a tomorrow. Aren't friendships also exercises in hope, in letting go, in acceptance? Don't they also help you to imagine exactly that future that you can no longer imagine in the face of the crushing reality of the world? Or at least allow us not to lose the sense that there can be such a future and that what we do does, in fact, matter, in the end, at least a little bit? I couldn't say whether I believed this – or whether I just wanted to.

The Kindness of Strangers

Pride assumes many forms. Some are beneficial. Others can represent an almost-insurmountable obstacle in one's life. I am rarely proud of my work, no matter how much agony it has cost me, no matter how hard I have toiled. I don't want to read my own writing after it has been published; or at least not for a few years, until it feels like it's been written by someone else. Until so much time has passed that, in some sense, it has, in fact, been written by someone else. I almost never manage to feel truly proud of the life I have built for myself, even though I've achieved some of the things I set out to achieve, even though I know how right that would be, not least as a sign of gratitude.

What I am also well aware of are the negative varieties of pride, those that consist of keeping your inner life under wraps, of not showing other people how you feel. Ignoring difficulties. Keeping your chin up and pushing on through. Keeping your composure. Which helps you keep your head above water when you're in difficult situations – or that's what I tell myself, at least. But at some point, that composure morphs into a constricting second skin. It becomes difficult to admit to yourself how you feel; you repress things and put things away again and again. And these things that, deep down, you somehow know but don't want to know – they begin to accumulate. So much so that the pressure of this knowledge becomes painful.

Am I too proud to admit to myself that I find my life alone more difficult than I would like to imagine it was? That I struggle with it more than I admit and that I actually wish that things were different? Am I, in other words, too proud to admit that I sometimes feel lonely?

Leafing through those same books that I return to time and time again, I come across sentences like this, which I have underlined: 'Today, it seems to him, that he writes more openly . . . He says this without the infatuation which may accompany all declarations of independence, and without the pose of melancholy adopted to avow a solitude.'[1] The sentences come from Roland Barthes' autobiographical book *On the Self and Writing*. I must have underlined these lines a long time ago. Still, I feel like I'm reading them for the first time.

As I flip through Maggie Nelson's *Bluets*, her reflections on the end of a love affair and the allure of the colour blue, the following sentence awaits me, highlighted in fading neon pink: 'I have been trying, for some time now, to find dignity in my loneliness. I have been finding this hard to do.'[2] The highlighted section is followed by three exclamation marks. There must have been a time when I could identify with Nelson's laconic lines. Do I still do so now?

And finally, opening Marguerite Duras' *Writing*, her essay on the loneliness of writers, I read: 'As soon as a human being is left alone, she tips into un-reason. I believe this: I believe that a person left to her own devices is already stricken by madness, because nothing keeps her from the sudden emergence of her personal delirium.'[3] When I read these lines, my heart beats a little faster. Involuntary waves of recognition under stirrings of resistance. Chin up, hold back, keep your cool.

I DIDN'T REALLY FEEL like going to Switzerland. A hotel in Lucerne had invited me to take part in a three-week writers' residency. After mulling it over for a while, I finally accepted. I needed time to write, I didn't know the Lake Lucerne region, and there was something soothing about the idea of escaping the grey Berlin January. But now my doubts had returned. I didn't want to see anyone, or even leave my flat, for that matter.

Part of the reason that the idea of the residency had originally appealed to me was because I had read Anita Brookner's novel *Hotel du Lac* a few months earlier and it had become one of my favourite books. A British friend of mine felt the same way, and in our conversations we kept coming back to that novel from the early 1980s. In it, the London-based protagonist, Edith Hope, a romance writer, is sent by her friends to an elegant, old-fashioned hotel on Lac Léman for an indefinite period of time in order to put an end to the risky and, to their mind, indecent affair she has been carrying on with a married man. At the centre of this astonishing book, which frustrates all of the classic narratives of traditional romance, is Edith having to confront her social status as a single woman about to turn forty. I couldn't say why I, as a gay man, found this novel so wonderful. Probably because it has such a dark centre and exposes, with such subtle humour, the multi-layered ways in which a society based on the institution of marriage excludes certain people. Despite all of her proclamations of fragility, Edith is an immensely strong person. She manages to create a space for herself in a society that intends to provide only a very narrowly defined place for her. I found that inspiring. And I kept thinking about Edith's stay in her elegant hotel, the big Swiss lake, the snow-covered mountains on the horizon.

I have always liked Switzerland. I'm usually in Zurich a couple of times a year for work. I wrote parts of my second book in Geneva.

I spent a summer in Lausanne with my former partner, David. Another man invited me to St Moritz a few years later, where we trudged through the snow to a dinner at the home of an art collector in whose living room hung the largest Basquiat I had ever seen. I had been to Basel to write about the art fair and in Valais to read at a literary festival.

The country sometimes seemed to me like the fulfilment of everything promised by the adverts I had marvelled at on West German television as a child. Everything is so clean and progressive and all in just the right measure, radiating the well-ordered glow of prosperity. I felt this, although I was aware that I was succumbing to a completely unwarranted idealization.

I USUALLY STRUGGLE at this time of year, so I should have known that it would be hard for me to get started. It had begun again a few weeks earlier, the feeling that always hits me at the end of a year. It sets in when the days become so short that I have to leave my desk no later than three o'clock so that I can still catch a little daylight on my daily walk through the park. When winter arrives, when my birthday approaches just before Christmas, when the festivities themselves begin, when one year changes to the next, when the months of darkness that follow don't seem to end – it is at this time that I feel, most powerfully, that I live alone.

The feeling is vague, when it begins. A certain kind of restlessness throughout my body, a desire that I cannot name, a yearning for something that I cannot identify. When I feel it, I work even harder, wander around town for even longer than usual, go to concerts, the ballet or the cinema more often, start reading a thick novel that I don't finish, look for the perfect Christmas presents for my godchildren, start to make marmalade from oranges or Meyer lemons to give away as gifts, make panettone and stollen for friends and eat more of it myself than I had planned to. For a few years now, I have put up a tree at the beginning of the festive period, obsessively decorating it with glittering baubles and ornaments until it resembles one of those luxurious Parisian dresses you see in paintings by John Singer Sargent or James Tissot. Today, the Christmas decorations pile up in my storeroom.

Sometimes all of this extra activity helps me, but sometimes it takes on a compulsive, manic quality and threatens to tip over into a mental state that is not yet depressive in itself, but can initiate a depression and, if I'm not careful, become so pervasive that it will dominate my life for weeks and months to come. At this stage, everything suddenly feels threadbare. Self-deceptions that have kept me afloat for most of the year begin to crumble away. The wilful oblivion on which most of our lives are based begins to fail. I can't describe it any better than that. It feels like the loss of an important fantasy. I stop believing that this life, as I live it, as I live it alone, is a good life.

This fantasy of a good life is more than just a personal fantasy of my own. It is a collective construct that many of us share, a fiction that is socially enacted and performed over and over again, by ourselves, by the people we love, by all of us. Even if you try to consciously detach yourself from it, you are confronted every day with the traces it has left behind in you. Part of this fiction consists in a complex illusion of affluence: the belief that we can make a good living based on our work, that with the necessary effort each and every one of us can achieve a certain degree of prosperity. Other aspects of this illusion include having a functioning romantic relationship, having a family of one's own, and these aspects often carry even more weight, not least because they are less questioned, because they take up a seemingly more natural place in the genetics of our social lives.

This fantasy construct of a good life represents a promise that we cling to despite the overwhelming evidence that for many of us it will never be fulfilled. According to the American philosopher Lauren Berlant, this clinging on often only puts obstacles in our way, because in the society in which we live – for many, if not most of us – it's not possible to lead this promised kind of life. Berlant has called this phenomenon 'cruel optimism'. For her, it is a signature of our age.[4] Sometimes, she writes, our everyday life feels like some sort of survival training that no longer allows us to plan realistically for the future, but only to fantasize about it.[5] This is not a pathology, she stresses, but an appropriate reaction to the world, a way of making life bearable, a life that confronts us again and again with contradictions, difficulties and ambivalence.[6]

The dark mood that recurs when each year comes to an end is, in large part, fed by my inner cruel optimism collapsing in the face of a frenetic celebration of the good life everywhere around me. I feel like I have failed. Because I don't have a partner, because my life as a writer is marked by financial insecurity. Everywhere I go, I am confronted with the fact that I have to make do without the two basic components of the good life as we imagine it: prosperity and happiness in love. I realize how cruel it really is to hold on to the belief that things will one day be different. I never feel as lonely as I do at the end of the year.

This loneliness has nothing to do with how I spend the holidays themselves. That year, I had also seen and spoken to friends, my parents and siblings. I spent Christmas Eve, as I often do, with Marie, one of my oldest friends; Olaf, her partner; and their son John, my godchild. On Christmas Day I was invited to a Mexican

Christmas lunch at Amy and Daniel's place, which was teeming with funny toddlers, and then I went to dinner at Karsten and Harriet's. I spent New Year's Eve at a party at Rabea and David's. My feeling of loneliness has nothing to do with whether or not I am actually alone. It is a seasonal loneliness, the symptom of a time in which I fail to make myself see what I usually see: that I may not be living a conventionally good life, but it is a full life, nonetheless, an exciting life, a life full of other kinds of prosperity and love.

I think a lot of people who live alone feel this way. As soon as the first Christmas lights appear on the streets, psychological dynamics are set into motion that are hard to escape. Instinctively, one feels as if one is moving through a world that belongs to other people, to lovers, to mothers and fathers, to grandparents. Roland Barthes described this feeling as a form of philosophical loneliness, a loneliness that arises because one moves outside of social systems and categories: 'Quite simply, I have no dialogue,' he writes in *A Lover's Discourse: Fragments*. 'In return, society subjects me to a strange, public repression: I am merely suspended, *a humanis*, far from human things, by a tacit decree of insignificance: I belong to no repertoire, participate in no asylum.'[7]

DESPITE MY END-OF-YEAR MOOD, I did travel to Lake Lucerne. It took some effort to make the travel arrangements, pack my suitcase and ask Tim, my neighbour, to empty my mailbox. But maybe the stay would do me good, I thought.

The hotel, called Beau Séjour, was situated directly on the lake and was even more charming than I had imagined. The two owners had done everything they could to live up to the promise of the hotel's name. I was touched by their generosity. They had set up a small office for me and had given me a room with a view of the lake and the mountains. From my bed, I could watch the sun rise in the morning. When I sat on the balcony and smoked – I still hadn't managed to quit, having taken it back up again four years earlier – I saw the big, white steamers sailing over the still water. I looked up at the sun-drenched winter sky and the snow-covered mountains, the Pilatus, the Bürgenstock, the Rigi, and couldn't believe how extraordinarily, how unimaginably beautiful the world could look. What solace.

I don't know why it was that I started hiking, but, to my surprise, I did. It must have been the sight of that enchanting landscape every day that made me want to go outside, right into the mountains, into the forest and the snow. But it probably also had something to do with the new, dangerous virus that had been discovered in Wuhan in China. Every day, in the news, I read about how first hundreds and then thousands of people had died from the pneumonia it caused. It still felt safe in Lucerne – only a few people there seemed to be concerned about it – but still I couldn't quite shake my anxiety. I needed to do something to quell my fears, sooth my nerves, make me feel alive.

I invested part of my stipend into buying a solid pair of hiking boots, merino wool shirts and a suitable outdoor jacket. While shopping, I met a friendly saleswoman who, in addition to the snow-covered winter hiking trails, recommended a few easy, lower-lying hiking routes where I would be able to test out my capabilities.

I THINK THAT WRITERS like walking so much because it is a good remedy for the dark state of mind that catches up with you, whether you like it or not, when you are working alone at your desk. It is not uncommonly the case that the great depressives of literary history have also been the most enthusiastic hikers. The list of writers who lifted their spirits by walking in nature is long: William and Dorothy Wordsworth, Henry David Thoreau, Robert Louis Stevenson, Goethe, of course, Rousseau, Nietzsche and many others. Michel de Montaigne loved to wander aimlessly through the idyllic landscape of Périgord; he was generally wary of meeting other people. For Virginia Woolf – the most gifted of novelists, the most gifted of hikers and, tragically, the most gifted of depressives – salvation lay in the hills of Sussex and along the cliffs of Cornwall. 'After the solitude of one's own room', she could only shed her 'self' by walking, she once explained.[8] I knew what she meant. She was not concerned with self-discovery. When you hike because you are not well, you don't want to find yourself. Or at least not at first. What you really want is to run away from yourself.

As it turned out, there is nowhere better to run away from yourself than in the mountains around Lake Lucerne. To begin with, I tried out hikes that didn't last longer than three or four hours. They were physically and mentally more challenging than I had expected. In the Alps, my northern German sense of heights transmuted, again and again, into a slightly queasy feeling. I got into some difficult situations that were so challenging from a hiking point of view that I didn't know what to do. But, eventually, I managed to meet these challenges. Every now and again another hiker I met on the trail would explain to me how to get down steep steps carved into the rock or a narrow slope that only seemed to be held together by a few tree roots. Sometimes I simply took a break and, afterwards, was able to find my own way down.

Soon, I found myself in the mountains on a regular basis, and I began to hike the easier sections of the Waldstätterweg, the trail around Lake Lucerne, that are open year-round. I would take a boat to the start of one of the hiking trails and walk for hours, always timing my return to catch the last boat back to town before dark. I had sore muscles and all kinds of aches and pains in my feet, legs, back and arms, yet, after a day or two back at my desk, I would set off again. The incredibly intense, life-affirming and liberating sunlight at higher altitudes, the ice-clear air, the snow, the cold on my face, it all made me feel euphoric in an unforeseen way, cleared my head so completely that I totally forgot about my life in Berlin. When you do nothing but put one foot in front of the other, your mind seems to seek new paths. Body, mind and world come together in a new way, open up new conversations. A very unique, rhythmic kind of thinking emerges, determined by the walking itself, by landscape and breath.[9]

With each hike, I had more faith in myself. Over and over again I savoured the beauty of the landscape; over and over again I reached my physical limits, coped with being alone in the vastness of nature; over and over again, I seemed, for a brief moment, to be able to see things differently, afresh. The movements of my body brought back memories of long-forgotten incidents from my past. Everything seemed to take on a larger and clearer context. Something was always at work within me. Without realizing it, I was thinking constantly about myself and my life. The mountains were so big, I was so small and so free of everything that actually determined my everyday life. I understood the enthusiasm with which people go hiking, I felt it anew each time.

SOON I BEGAN TO FEEL a little better. The hiking certainly had a big part to play in this. The luxury of having a room with a view, an office just for work, and the fact that, for weeks at the hotel, I barely had to worry about the everyday trivialities of life. But the biggest influence on my mood were, surprisingly, the people who worked at the Beau Séjour. The owners had mainly employed friends or people they knew well, so that life in the hotel exuded a sense of something communal, something familiar, and after a few days it was clear to me that, without being able to say why, I liked almost all of them. There was something idiosyncratic about it; it was a spontaneous liking, a reflexive concord that came with the knowledge that we saw things in a similar way, shared certain reference points in this chaotic world, certain sympathies, certain aversions. These kinds of 'spontaneous alliances', as the literary critic Silvia Bovenschen once called them, are of course not really reliable. But they are beautiful, because they are so fleeting and do sometimes spark the beginning of a real friendship.[10]

The truth is that even relationships that we would not initially describe as being intimate or close have a significance for us and our internal sense of harmony. Not only do we live within a close circle of friends, family members and partners, but we move in much wider social circles. These 'networks', if you want to call them that, are often hard to grasp, but, generally speaking, they have a far greater influence on our everyday life than we think.[11]

The first person to study this phenomenon was the sociologist Mark S. Granovetter. In his essay 'The Strength of Weak Ties', written in the early 1970s, he expressed something that had previously been understood only intuitively, at best. Whether it is acquaintances, neighbours, colleagues, friends of friends, people we only meet by chance or on certain occasions, Granovetter believed that there is great strength in these 'weak social ties'. For him, these relationships fulfil a certain 'bridging function' and are predestined to pass on information that cannot be passed on in any other way.[12] A number of social scientists have taken up the mantle of his research and demonstrated how easily ideas, mindsets, attitudes, fashions, feelings and affects, such as confidence and fear, spread in these networks, and how much we are shaped by them, without ever realizing it.[13]

One facet in particular of my new little 'network' that did me a world of good during my time on Lake Lucerne was a fundamental and judicious kindness that I often miss in everyday life in Berlin. Kindness is something that some people are suspicious of, believing it to be either boring or insincere. There seems to be something antiquated about the idea, something stiff and anachronistic that runs counter to the neoliberal spirit of our day. When, as a matter of course, societies divide their members into winners and losers, this leads, perhaps inevitably, to people only being kind if they need to be.

But, as psychoanalyst Adam Phillips and cultural historian Barbara Taylor write in their book *On Kindness*, though it has acquired the status of a 'forbidden pleasure' in recent decades, kindness is something that 'remains essential to our emotional and mental health'. Phillips and Taylor are thinking both about what it is like to experience other people's kindness and what it is like to be kind to other people. And they mean ordinary kindness in our everyday lives. According to their observations, it is this very kindness that is repeatedly defined as a sign of weakness, which, in turn, makes us avoid being kind and then find all sorts of justifications for doing so.[14]

Sometimes you're sitting on the bus or the train and you have the impression that the flood of hateful online comments, devoid of any self-reflection, has spilled over into the real world. Most of us know how painful careless judgements, inattentiveness and microaggressions can be. Nevertheless, for a lot of people, being kind seems to represent a real challenge. In part, this stems from a form of cultural conditioning. In Germany, for instance, being 'direct' and able to speak 'uncomfortable' truths is deemed, by many, to be something positive. But one could also ask oneself, of course, whether one's own assessment of a given situation is in fact so important that one is happy to hurt someone else in order to express it. It is not uncommon for the expression of so-called uncomfortable truths to conceal a certain kind of comfort: one's own unwillingness to muster even a modicum of empathy.

It is not difficult to be kind. Usually, it is one of the first intuitive reactions we have when we encounter other people. It is not difficult to show a little interest in someone else, to listen, not difficult to realize that we are all vulnerable, that what we say has consequences and that we are often wrong precisely in our conviction that we are right.[15]

I have hurt many people in my life, sometimes intentionally, but also involuntarily when I have failed to be considerate. And, of course, I have also experienced many such grievances myself. I don't know if I always succeed in being kind, but at least I try. You never know what's going on behind the facade that the other person presents to you, you never know what other people's lives are like, what they have to deal with every day. From the outside, people almost always appear stronger than they feel on the inside.

IT TOOK A WHILE before I really felt better again. Until I no longer felt so keenly the inherent cruelty of my optimistic fantasies about the good life. Until the things that I didn't want to know about actually became things that I didn't know about again, or at least things that I didn't know that much about. Until the necessary self-deception on which life is based started to function properly again. That January was to become the first New Year in a long time that didn't begin with me battling a depressive episode. At some point, being alone no longer hurt; at some point, I no longer felt alone.

Towards the end of my stay, after a hike, I sat on the outer deck of one of the boats back to Lucerne. It was very cold, but I wrapped myself up in a big scarf and watched the play of the waves, watched the mute swans, the great crested grebes and red-crested pochards glide across the water, watched the mountains and the villages pass me by with their picturesque churches, elegant houses and grand hotels from the nineteenth century, which looked as if another era was living on inside of them. Suddenly I saw the words 'Hotel du Lac' on one of these magnificent buildings. My heart leapt. I took a photo and sent it to the friend I had been talking to about Anita Brookner's novel. I knew it would make him smile. Edith Hope, I should say, decides at the end of the book to leave the man she is having an affair with and probably loves. But she also rejects the man who, with little emotion, offers her his hand in marriage – a marriage that in and of itself would represent social inclusion and recognition. She decides to live alone.

Living alone presents challenges that are incomprehensible to people with partners, spouses and families. Even people in a relationship can feel lonely, but if you live alone and feel lonely, you will stay that way for the foreseeable future. Loneliness ebbs and flows; sometimes it is an acute feeling, then it is forgotten, or it is easily pushed aside until it hits you again. Regardless of whether you live alone by choice or not, regardless of how many friends you have, regardless of how well you organize your life. Loneliness is sometimes a corollary of living alone. How difficult it is to accept that.

It is always easier to convince oneself that one does not feel the pain – which one hopes, out of pride, to hide from the world – than to actually look that pain in the eye and grapple with it. But all feelings, good and bad, have to be felt, accepted and lived through. Sometimes living alone hurts, sometimes it doesn't. Sometimes you have to find new ways of coping, or at least be open to the possibility of new ways. Sometimes you have to dare yourself to go out onto the lake and into the mountains, to hold your face up to the winter sun and hold on to all those kind people who are accompanying you for part of your journey. And to remember that there are not only different kinds of pride, but also different kinds of solitude. And yes, different kinds of loneliness.

Conversations
with Friends

When I returned to Berlin, I did not yet know we were at the beginning of a period that, for many people, would mean the end of normality. This ending had, in fact, been foreseen for several years. The process had been underway for some time, but people had become so accustomed to it that its momentum was barely noticed. The virus that I had been so afraid of in Lucerne was spreading inexorably around the world. And everyone was surprised by what should not have been a surprise, given the course of the disease, the incidence rates and the number of infections reported in China. Many scientists had been warning for years that the destruction of natural habitats, factory farming and global mobility would increase the likelihood of zoonotic viral diseases. Now, these warnings had become a reality.

A few days after I'd returned from Switzerland, I fell ill. What felt like a normal flu or cold that it took me a month to shake off was probably just that: a normal flu or cold. I often suffer from these kinds of infections in winter, but the general sense of uncertainty all around me and the fact that, at that time, it was not yet possible to be tested for the new virus made me cautious. I kept to my flat, hardly saw anyone, and the few times I did, it was only outdoors for short walks. I was in contact with most of the people in my life virtually or by phone. When I wasn't working, I was reading.

I HAVE SOME FRIENDS who I have known for over two decades. These friendships were forged in my first university course in Berlin, in the Department for Comparative Literature, which, back at the tail end of the nineties, was still located in a sleepy villa in the suburb of Dahlem. When I think back to the beginnings of those relationships, I realize that they almost all arose from precisely those idiosyncratic 'spontaneous alliances' that Silvia Bovenschen described, coupled with a degree of serendipity. For a long time, friendship seemed to me to be primarily a question of identification. A question of mutual recognition in emotional conversations, in the exchange of thoughts and ideas about the world, a shared recognition that, during long evenings spent together, would often take on an intoxicating quality.

The subject of the undergraduate class that I met many of these friends on was 'Narcissism and Doppelgangers'. The amount of reading we were allocated for the course was so intimidating that it left many of us speechless, not only due to the volume of texts we had to read but also how demanding they were. The course required us to read Ovid's *Metamorphoses*, psychoanalytical essays by Sigmund Freud and Jacques Lacan, E.T.A. Hoffmann's *The Devil's Elixirs*, Jean Paul's *Siebenkäs*, Kafka's *Metamorphosis*, an old French drama the title of which I can't now recollect because I never read it, nor many of the other books we were allocated. The real kicker was that the reading lists contained only texts in the original language. Naturally, one was expected to read Ovid in the original Latin and that play in Old French. Except for those people who were blessed with an unshakeable self-confidence, almost all of us were pretty much at a loss. It was an experience that welded some of us together as we searched in libraries for translations and explanatory secondary literature. We were all new to Berlin. Everything seemed exciting. It was a time of new beginnings.

Despite the importance of my friends in my life, I feel reticent about the increasingly prominent celebration of friendship over the last few years, and I can't quite put my finger on why. There seems to be some sort of collective need to engage with the topic, as evidenced by the success of often well-written, edifying books such as Dolly Alderton's *Everything I Know about Love* and Aminatou Sow and Ann Friedman's *Big Friendship*. Popular science books, such as Lydia Denworth's *Friendship* or Nicholas A. Christakis's *Blueprint*, are also part of this conversation. Even classic self-help guides to friendship, like Dale Carnegie's *How to Win Friends and Influence People*, continue to enjoy a surprisingly unreserved popularity. At their core, these texts always say the same thing. They are variations on a 'celebration of friendship', a classic topos in the history of philosophy and literature. They almost always explain how important friendship is for a good life, for our happiness and for our mental health. And they almost always describe a range of particularly moving scenes from intimate friendships.

There is often something strangely saccharine about this celebration, not least because it is limited to variations on a somewhat trite ideal of friendship that reflects a 'catalogue of highly old-fashioned virtues', as Silvia Bovenschen puts it. 'Loyalty, truthfulness, faithfulness' are among them, 'but also discretion, respect, distance, independence, tact, taste (the list goes on)'.[1] Within this framework, friendships usually take the form of a kind of therapeutic *deus ex machina* that solves every kind of life problem – a quick and obtainable consolation prize for anyone left alone. When every other tether to love has been broken, there seem to be friendships waiting for you, your own little substitute for happiness.

Why are we, as a culture, revisiting this classic topos: the celebration of friendship? At a time in which the fundamental inequalities in our society are becoming ever more apparent, a time characterized by experiences of contingency, precarious ways of living and a fear of the future, and in which interpersonal bonds seem more fragile than ever? Can this new paean not also be understood as another facet of Lauren Berlant's cruel optimism? As a form of a certain kind of magical thinking? Has friendship become one of the straws that we grasp at while the world collapses around us?

MOST OF THE PUBLICATIONS touched on above represent a continuation of a long cultural history of the philosophical idealization of amicable relationships, stretching back to ancient Greece. Almost all of the great philosophers of antiquity, from Plato, Aristotle and Epicurus to Cicero, Seneca and Plutarch, left behind teachings on friendship. For these scholars, friendships were part of the true eudaemonia, of the happy life, the very project of philosophy.[2] It was therefore no coincidence that 'philosophy' already contained the ancient Greek term for friendship: *philia*.[3] As Gilles Deleuze and Félix Guattari pointed out, it was the very notion of friendship that provided the dialogic of thought. It was the foundation of philosophical competition and created the very conditions that made it possible for one to deal with the rivalry of one's competitors.[4]

Books VIII and IX of Aristotle's *Nicomachean Ethics*, penned in the fourth century BC, belong to those texts of human history that, when we read them, remind us of the degree to which they continue to shape our culture to this day. Aristotle not only described friendship as one of life's greatest gifts and highest virtues, but, by and large, he also concealed the more challenging and darker aspects of this kind of relationship.[5] In doing so, as the philosopher Alexander Nehamas explains, Aristotle established something of a philosophical tradition. It was Aristotle, for example, who originated the idea that friendship exists when the well-being of another person is as important to us as our own well-being and that this goodwill is based on reciprocity.[6] He also introduced the idea of self-friendship or self-love as being a basic prerequisite for becoming friends with other people – a notion echoed in modern therapeutic conceptions of self-confidence, self-respect and self-worth.[7]

One of the pillars of Aristotelian thought on friendship is the idea of how alike friends are, an idea expressed in the occasionally jubilant way in which I identified with the friends I met on my first university course. Ever since Aristotle's *Nicomachean Ethics*, friendship has been defined as a relationship between like-minded people – between people who perceive the world in the same way, have had similar life experiences and have the same political opinions, people with a similar psychological and emotional make-up and similar personal histories. True friendship, according to Aristotle, is based on 'equality and agreement', on finding ourselves in the other and vice versa, on the fact that the 'friend' is 'a second, separate self'.[8]

Towards the end of the sixteenth century, Michel de Montaigne emphatically brought this ideal of friendship into the modern age. In his essay *On Friendship* – to this day, one of the most widely read and cited texts on the subject – he wrestled with finding an appropriate form to write about the death of his beloved friend Étienne de La Boétie. He succeeded in doing so by liberating the idea of friendship, refashioned in the Middle Ages through Christian ideas of loving God and thy neighbour, and applying it again to a relationship between two people. Intimate friendship, and not the confessional, was for Montaigne, the space in which nothing should remain unsaid.[9]

In some ways, Montaigne further radicalized the egalitarian dimension of Aristotelian thinking on friendship. He regarded the friend as an alter ego, a person in whom he realized himself. It was only in Montaigne's work that Aristotle's unification fantasy came fully to fruition: 'But in the friendship I speak of', he writes, their two souls 'mix and work themselves into one piece, with so universal a mixture, that there is no more sign of the seam by which they were first conjoined.'[10] This ecstatic ideal of friendship is expressed in an almost exuberant language of love: 'Our souls had drawn so unanimously together, they had considered each other with so ardent an affection, and with the like affection laid open the very bottom of our hearts to one another's view', Montaigne says of Boétie, 'that I not only knew his as well as my own; but should certainly in any concern of mine have trusted my interest much more willingly with him, than with myself.'[11]

To borrow an image from the philosopher Jacques Derrida, Aristotle's and Montaigne's historical texts could be described as two powerful earthquakes in our understanding of friendship.[12] Two earthquakes that have thrown up the terrain on which we walk today when we think about and practise friendship. Regardless of whether the ideal sketched out in these texts stretches the limits of what is actually possible in a friendship, regardless of whether it ensures that every real-life friendship seems highly deficient in comparison.

How problematic this emphatic idea of sameness this 'friend as "another oneself"' is in philosophical terms is outlined by Derrida in his influential book *The Politics of Friendship*. According to Derrida, most classical discourses on friendship focus on a person merging with another into an identical (and same-sex) double. They focus on '*homogeneity*', '*homophilia*' and an 'affinity (*bebaion*) stemming from birth, from native community'.[13]

The fact that this classical understanding of friendship meant, of course, only friendships between wealthy, heterosexual and, of course, white men is not just a historical footnote. Philosophical thinking around friendship that focuses on sameness is, in the end, always an expression of what female philosophers and psychoanalysts such as Luce Irigaray, Hélène Cixous and Julia Kristeva have so aptly called 'phallogocentrism'. In a way, you might even say that it's one of its foundations. 'Phallogocentrism' is an understanding of the world based on a purely heterosexual, male perspective. For neither Aristotle nor Montaigne did friendships exist between men and women or between women and women. Both believed that only upper-class men had the intellectual capacity to maintain friendships. This belief persisted into twentieth-century philosophy and is still echoed today in ideas of male-only or female-only friendships.

They should have known better. Two hundred and fifty years before Aristotle, the poet Sappho was writing poems in Mytilene on Lesbos that were not only about love but also about friendship. Four hundred years before Montaigne, the letters of the polymath Hildegard von Bingen testified to the deep friendships that developed between nuns in convents. Women in the Beguine orders of the Middle Ages and in Renaissance high society often struck up public friendships with other women. At the end of the sixteenth century, the Venetian writer Moderata Fonte composed dialogues in which she argued, among other things, that women were far more capable of forming and maintaining friendships than men.[14]

And this was before the eighteenth century, often considered to be the 'century of friendship' because of its almost cult-like veneration of the figure of the friend; before Jane Austen went on to explore complex heterosocial friendships in her novels;[15] before the emergence of the phenomenon of 'romantic friendship', a form of friendship between women that, with its confessions of love and vows of fidelity, drew on classical notions of romantic love, but in which this romantic love was not usually consummated sexually. Reading the correspondences between Madame de Staël and Madame Récamier or Emily Dickinson and her sister-in-law Sue Gilbert would convince anyone of the power these friendships could have.[16]

Western intellectual history has ignored, belittled or ridiculed all friendships between people who are not upper-class white heterosexual men, an assertion of power that runs counter to all available evidence on the subject. Perhaps because it secretly recognized the threat to patriarchal domination that these friendships posed, perhaps because it intuitively recognized the explosive power of a way of thinking about friendship that was not based on equality but instead celebrated the diversity of life.

THAT INTRODUCTORY COURSE on 'Narcissism and Doppelgangers' was, in many ways, one of the most influential classes I have ever taken. It delved into a long literary and philosophical history of self-mirroring, a history of all the wrong paths people take when they are unable to break through the limits of how they view themselves and the world, a history of the impenetrable barriers created when people only search, in other people, for what they already know. Even though I still haven't managed to read Lacan in

French, I have often returned to many of the texts discussed in that course. They informed my thinking during my studies and beyond, so much so that when I knew I wanted to undertake psychoanalysis, it was the Lacanian style of psychoanalysis that I picked.

I also thought back about that course when I read a study about the friendships that arose among the students of an introductory psychology course at the University of Leipzig. The researchers of that study discovered that, contrary to what they believed, the students became friends with each other not so much because of how similar their personalities were, but simply because they were assigned to the same group. If the students sat in the same row during a given lecture, the likelihood that they would become friends greatly increased. And this was most likely to happen when they actually sat next to each other. It turned out that, when it came to making friends, accidental physical proximity trumped all other cards.[17]

A similar study at Utrecht University found that the archetype of the alter ego does indeed play a role in who we choose to be friends with, but in a completely different way than had been previously thought. In order to become friends, the students in Utrecht did not have to resemble each other at all. Instead, they perceived themselves as being similar even when they were not. They succumbed to their narcissistic desire for recognition and mirroring. They only felt that they had met like-minded people in whom they recognized themselves and saw themselves reflected.[18]

This myth of harmony between friends is occasionally perpetuated even by the natural sciences. According to one paper, pairs of friends perceive the world in a neurologically similar way and interpret it similarly. The assumption here is that these similarities are a given from the outset and are not the result of a sustained dialogue, of togetherness, a shared life. The paper even claimed that there was a certain genetic similarity found between pairs of friends, although the author himself had to admit that the results require closer examination and that the similarity in question is vanishingly small. And yet, in nearly all of the recent articles, podcasts and books on the subject of friendship that cite it, this qualification is missing.[19] The promise of a seemingly simple answer to the complex question of why people are friends with other people seems to just be too tempting. Unintentionally, this research, and especially the questions underlying it, ultimately illustrate only how profoundly our current understanding of friendship is shaped by notions of self-mirroring.

WHEN I LOOK BACK at the friendships I made in that literature course, I realize that this feeling of identifying with one another is rarely a good indicator of how long these friendships would last and how important they would become for me. In the long run, in our friends, it is not a wise strategy to seek out doppelgangers – on the contrary, in fact. Most friendships only survive the passing of time, the shifting phases of life, the changing locations, attitudes and personal constellations when you leave behind this narcissistic desire to recognize yourself in the person sitting in front of you. The friends from that time in my life that I am still close to today are those with whom I have succeeded in doing just that.

More recently, philosophers like Alexander Nehamas have suggested that we should try to understand friendships as 'organisms', as something living that emerges from the interplay of interdependent organs. This is a beautiful image. Friendships can flourish, but they can also fall apart. For them to last, you have to talk to each other, have shared experiences, relate to each other emotionally, you have to rid yourself of the notion of the alter ego. If we fail to do this, we turn our friends into 'objects of friendship' and thus destroy the basic prerequisite of every friendship: real personal involvement, that 'special form of togetherness' in a friendship, its 'being together-ness', its 'we-ness', as the philosopher Klaus-Dieter Eichler calls it. It is so easy to succumb to the temptation to understand friends as part of and as an extension of oneself, to love them because of their supposed similarity to one's own self.[20] But the calculation of sameness and the narcissistic appropriation that it entails ultimately constitute a form of involuntary violence. You necessarily misjudge the other. You miss the chance to find out who this person you are close to really is.

BUT WHAT MIGHT friendships look like if they were not sustained by this ideal of the like-minded friend? Philosophers such as Hannah Arendt reflected on this question, and she had many such friendships herself. For her, the power and significance of this form of relationship lay precisely in its lived pluralistic practice.[21] Her friends included well-known intellectuals on two continents: Martin Heidegger, Mary McCarthy, Uwe Johnson, Alfred Kazin and Karl Jaspers. She maintained lively contact with them, in person, by letter and telephone, and regularly visited her European friends after emigrating to New York at the end of the war at considerable personal logistical and financial expense. Even when she disagreed with them politically and ideologically, she remained loyal.[22]

Hannah Arendt found a champion for her understanding of friendship in Gotthold Ephraim Lessing, as she wrote in her speech 'On Humanity in Dark Times: Thoughts about Lessing'. In the well-known 'ring parable', central to his play *Nathan the Wise*, Lessing illustrated that all three world religions and, at the same time, none of them can lay claim to sovereignty over the truth. In the parable, a ring that renders the bearer pleasing in the eyes of God has been passed down the generations. But when a father cannot choose between his three sons, he has two replicas made. The sons learn that the only way of knowing if they had the real ring would be to live a life that honours God; as such, the authenticity of the ring would no longer matter. According to Arendt, Nathan's wisdom, his love of humanity and his openness to the world were based, above all, on the fact that he placed friendship above truth. Lessing, according to Arendt, would, without hesitation, sacrifice truth, even if it actually existed, 'to humanity, to the possibility of friendship and of discourse among men'. What distinguishes him is not merely the insight that there cannot be one single truth, but rather the fact that he was happy that it did not exist, because only in this way would 'the discourse among men' never cease.[23]

The pivotal point of Arendt's lived philosophy of friendship was thus the recognition of the otherness of the other. For her, it was the differences between people, and not their sameness, that led to real friendship, to what takes place between the self and the other, to that in-betweenness in which a genuine exchange of experiences and views can take place, in which openness and mutual trust prevail, but in which, simultaneously, we are also able to experience alienation and reticence.[24]

As such, Arendt was anticipating the discourses of Post-Structuralist philosophers such as Emmanuel Lévinas, Jacques Derrida and Alain Badiou, each of whom attempted, in his own particular way, to do philosophical justice to 'the other'. Lévinas built an entire architecture of philosophy around the eternal nature of the other, on the fact that they can never be fully recognized and understood by the self. It was precisely from the point of view of this other that he tried to understand the world. Derrida, on the other hand, struck a gentler tone. Friendship, for him, was, by definition, about granting the other a place beyond the reach of one's own will. I often find myself reflecting on a line from Derrida's book on friendship. 'I renounce you, I have decided to,' the philosopher writes, is 'the most beautiful and the most inevitable . . . declaration of love'.[25]

DOESN'T THIS ALSO EXPLAIN the unease that I felt about the flood of publications in praise of the joy of friendships? I had the impression that this new emphatic celebration of friendship was the product of a cultural notion that is only realized, in our real relationships, in the briefest of flashes, and is the product of the inflated ideals of friendship that we invoke even though we secretly know that they have a tendency to evaporate whenever they are invoked. These conceptions of friendship arise from a timid view of life, a view that suppresses reality in service of a world of fantasy: the fantasy of total agreement, of self-affirmation, of relationships in which conflict is nominal.

Ideas like these appear to make our lives a little easier; they give us something to hold on to. But, at heart, they reflect the totalitarian desire for the 'one' opinion or the 'one' truth – which is of course one's own. True dialogue, as Hannah Arendt would say, the most constitutive element of our friendships, is made virtually impossible by these kinds of ideals. Friendship can only emerge when we meet each other again and again with openness and get to know each other from different sides. A friendship is 'newly "made", newly mixed . . . newly invented in each and every conversation', writes Silvia Bovenschen. Precisely therein lies its precarious beauty; precisely therein lies the strength of its bonds.

The joy of friendship cannot be located in its ideal. It does not materialize when the only thing being met is our own need for other people's attention. It does not transpire when we project our feelings and our unresolved conflicts onto our friends, or simply believe that the reason we know them so well is because they are so much like ourselves. The lasting joy of friendship is a by-product of giving, of gifting our attention. It is an experience of dissolving our barriers and occurs only when we succeed in broadening our own horizons and escaping the prison of our own problems and fears that we are so often trapped in. It materializes when we recognize the person in front of us in their otherness. When we open ourselves up to their emotional reality, to their alternative view of the world. It emerges when we are there for someone else.

Only the mutual recognition of each other's otherness ensures that relationships grow, that one grows oneself and that life liberates itself from the constraints of one's own necessarily limited fantasies. Friends help us to break through our narcissistic inner barrier and to perceive the whole reality of life. Without friends, it would be impossible to evolve, impossible to be truly human.

WHEN I LOOK AROUND at the friendships in my life, they are as diverse as the people I am friends with. As beautiful and limited, as loving and cool, as exciting and boring, as eye-opening and infuriating. None of them corresponds to the ideal of sameness; none of them is harmonious without fail. The semantics of friendship and its old-fashioned ideals become insignificant in the presence of real relationships. There are simply no rules, implicit or explicit statutes, no contracts, no sanctioning authorities, no external constraints when it comes to friendships. There is only me, the other person and what happens between us. Friendships are woven into our lives as perfectly and imperfectly as only real things can be.

In those weeks in which I was ill and which were spent largely alone in my flat, with books and my writing, I felt less alive. But the conversations between me and the people in my life did not stop. Conversations in which they were both distant and close to me at the same time, in which I could catch a glimpse of their view of the world. I could seek out closeness and know that there were people who had a stake in my life. To my own surprise, I did not feel lonely and, in a way, not even alone.

Never So Lonely

At some point in our lives, most of us reach a moment in which we realize that all is not what we once imagined it would be. A point at which certain convictions are shattered, dark premonitions come true and the sudden understanding that we are experiencing what seems like a watershed sends waves of disbelief rippling through our bodies. When the pandemic reached its peak in Berlin, it was precisely this feeling that I was gripped by.

In retrospect, I can't say why the situation felt so unreal to me for so long; I suspect that my psyche was protecting me from genuinely comprehending what was happening around me. It wasn't until a dinner with Jenny, a friend of mine who is a professor, that this changed. We have known each other since our student days, when, as PhD students, we shared an office and went out together in the evenings. Before we met up, we had assured each other that we were symptom-free and, initially, we talked about other things. But afterwards, as we walked through Moabit in the dark of the evening, she told me that her wife's sister, a nurse at Berlin's Charité hospital, was convinced that it was going to be as bad everywhere as it had been in China, and that no one in Germany was prepared for an epidemic of that magnitude. You have to be ready to go into quarantine overnight, she said, and you should definitely have enough food in your flat to last for at least two weeks.

Jenny sent me a text message the next day reminding me to buy supplies. When I went to the supermarket around the corner, I was dumbfounded to find that many of the shelves were empty. There was no flour or sugar left, nor any pasta, lentils, yeast or toilet paper. I assumed that this was only temporary and, to begin with, I wasn't worried at all. In my cupboards at home, I still had enough flour for the sourdough bread I baked for myself every week; I still had a bag of Puy lentils, a couple of boxes of good pasta and decent Italian canned tomatoes. But the longer I looked at the empty shelves, the more queasy I began to feel. It seemed to me as if a new film had begun, as if another narrative had taken over the reality of my life – the narrative of the apocalypse. The equilibrium of my social life suddenly seemed incredibly precarious. If people's solidarity was already failing in the comparatively relaxed situation we found ourselves in and they were already buying a year's supply of flour out from under other people's noses, then what was going to happen if there was a real catastrophe? There, in that supermarket, of all places, I was struck by the realization that, from this moment on, I was completely on my own. It felt as if I had been dealt a heavy blow.

EVEN THOUGH FEELINGS of loneliness are part of a life lived alone, that life does not necessarily have to be a lonely one. I am not afraid of being alone. Although I do sometimes struggle with it, it generally doesn't feel like a privation, but something that I enjoy. I like being home. I have a beautiful apartment that corresponds to my aesthetic ideas. I enjoy following the seasonal changes of my daily rhythms and not having to account for them to anyone. Of course, I love spending time with the people in my life. But I also enjoy the time I have to myself.

Like many things, this might stem from my childhood. I grew up in a big family in the countryside, where there was always something going on. There could be joy in that, but the greatest pleasure for me was to block out everything around me, to read or to walk alone in the forest or around the lake with our dog, lost in thought, for hours on end. The older I got, the more writing began to fill those hours. It was as if being alone distanced me a little from the world while simultaneously fashioning a new connection to it.

Later, in my twenties, I would completely unlearn this ability. For a long time I couldn't be alone without being seized by a vehement restlessness that I could only soothe by going out, by meeting people, by drinking, partying and flirting. This went on for many years, and, if I hadn't stopped drinking, it might have gone on like that for a few more – until at some point nothing much would have been going on at all. It was only then, when I had stopped drinking, that I learned to appreciate being alone again. Today, my everyday life is generally determined by a fundamental sense of not having enough time alone to myself, having too little time for the many things I want to do, too little time for the books I want to read, the exhibitions I want to see, the concerts and operas I want to go to, the films and series I want to watch. Too little time for the recipes I want to try out, the walks I want to take, the books I want to write.

But the pandemic knocked my life alone completely out of balance. The more it progressed, the more I began to feel a kind of solitude descending on me that I hadn't experienced before, even during my worst depressive episodes. I had the impression that I had never been so lonely.

LONELINESS MEANS SOMETHING different to each and every one of us. Some people are rarely haunted by it, others often are. We all feel it differently and each of us has our own way of dealing with it. Some people feel lonely after just a few evenings spent alone, others need only minimal social contact. But no one can be lonely for long periods without being damaged by it. Acute, prolonged loneliness creates, in most of us, an emotional hunger, a serious mental anguish accompanied by a marked loss of meaning and self-worth, with feelings of shame, guilt and despair. In addition to the sense of distance from other people that loneliness entails, it also entails a bewildering distance from oneself, from those sides of the self that exist only in connection with other people. Sometimes it feels as if one is experiencing a psychological breakdown. But loneliness is not a disease, it is a feeling – a complex feeling, but a feeling nevertheless. It is an important distinction.[1]

As the Norwegian philosopher Lars Svendsen demonstrates in his book *A Philosophy of Loneliness*, the current preoccupation with loneliness and the frequent invocation of a 'loneliness epidemic' is characterized by a fundamental misunderstanding: that the increasing number of people living alone in Western societies automatically means that more people must feel lonely. But 'being alone and being lonely', Svendsen says, 'are logically and empirically independent from each other'.[2] While there is indeed a statistical correlation between the phenomena of living alone and of loneliness, its magnitude and significance are usually overestimated. From the 1950s onwards, sociologists and journalists have been regularly trumpeting the emergence of a 'new loneliness', while lamenting the decline of traditional forms of social cohesion, even though there is little statistical evidence to support this beyond the fact that a growing number of people live by themselves.[3] Loneliness, in other words, cannot be diagnosed on the basis of the absence of a romantic relationship; the many other social ties in our lives are also capable of satisfying our need for intimacy.

I don't mean to suggest that social isolation is not a problem for many people. It is largely undisputed that it can lead to serious physical and mental problems.[4] The Harvard Grant Study, for example – a long-term sociological study that has been tracking the mental and physical health of several hundred Harvard graduates and their children since 1938 – leaves no doubt that close interpersonal relationships are one of the main predictors of a good life. People without these kinds of relationships get sick more often and usually die earlier than people with a fulfilling social life.[5] So I am not for a second suggesting that it is not important to talk about loneliness. On the contrary, talking about it can alleviate the shame associated with it, can ease the pain of it and help people who feel lonely understand that they are by no means alone in this.

But, often, these discussions about the 'loneliness epidemic' simply mask a wistful longing for the good old times, for traditional social models of marriage and family that for many of us have outlived their relevance. Often, behind these discussions, is a political agenda that fails to recognize our social realities. Significantly, each revival of the prophets of social decline fails to propose that we start fighting loneliness by tackling racism, misogyny, ableism, antisemitism, homo-, trans- and Islamophobia, by addressing the social stigmatization of people living in poverty, all the structural phenomena of exclusion that produce social isolation every day and on a vast scale. The response of those who employ these grand warnings is almost always to invoke the magical power of the nuclear family.

APPEALING TO OUR nostalgic inclinations is simple. The impulse
to portray loneliness as a pathological consequence of social change
likely masks a certain kind of defensiveness. It is a feeling that we do
not want to be responsible for, a feeling that we would rather not
have anything to do with. In her groundbreaking book *The Lonely
City*, the writer Olivia Laing describes the extensive social taboos
surrounding loneliness. Loneliness, she explains, runs so contrary
to the life we should be leading that most of us struggle to even
admit that we feel it.[6] Intuitively, we all have a sense of this taboo.
In our collective image of loneliness, there is always the suggestion
that the lonely deserve their fate, that they are too unattractive, shy,
solitary and self-centred, too prone to self-pity and complain too
much about their lot without any sense of dignity.[7] No one wants
to be like that.

This taboo not only permeates our social lives, it is also reflected
in our language, for example in the distinction between the words
'loneliness' and 'solitude' that exist in both German and English.
'Solitude' often comes across as the presentable, dignified version
of loneliness, like a kind of social isolation with little psychological
suffering. Many people almost reflexively refer to this distinction
when talking about loneliness. And it is precisely this reflexivity
that sometimes conceals a lingering feeling of shame. A shame that
prevents people from expressing their feelings of loneliness. I am
solitary, not lonely, they seem to say. I will not profess to you that
I am lonely. I am not vulnerable. My solitude does not hurt, I am
not suffering. And I don't want to be exposed to your vulnerability
either. It reminds me too much of my own. Please tell me this is
solitude, not loneliness.

Psychologists, such as Frieda Fromm-Reichmann, have researched
this force field of loneliness and its unsettling effect on other people.

Her essay 'Loneliness' from 1959, which also informed Olivia Laing's reflections, is considered one of the very first intellectual and psychiatric investigations of loneliness. In her essay, Fromm-Reichmann makes it clear that loneliness is often such a traumatic experience for us that we are simply not capable of feeling empathy for the lonely person, even if, theoretically, we should know how it feels to be lonely. We usually so successfully compartmentalize the memory of our own experiences of loneliness that they no longer even exist for us.[8]

The psychologist Robert Weiss observed this same phenomenon in his patients. Many people underestimate the role that loneliness plays in their lives, he writes in his book *Loneliness*, and they do so to a considerable degree. Even if the repressive mechanisms at work are not consistently successful, Weiss says, they still result in our inability to remember the intensity of our own experiences of loneliness. Accordingly, we are not able to imagine how painful this experience is for other people.

These avoidance strategies can even influence the psychotherapeutic process, Fromm-Reichmann noted. Loneliness, she writes, evokes a specific fear in the other person, a fear of contagion, from which even therapists cannot free themselves. The result is that many people, even if they suffer from relatively mild forms of loneliness, rarely get the chance to talk about it. Feeling lonely becomes an anxiety-ridden secret that cannot be adequately communicated.[9]

THE FURTHER THE YEAR progressed, the more I felt that my life alone with its occasional feelings of loneliness was now becoming a life that was fundamentally and permanently characterized by them. I wondered whether most people living alone were not also finding the developments of that year particularly challenging. The creeping anxiety about the future, the collective panic that kept breaking through, the news of illness and death that soon became part of our daily lives, and of course all of the social distancing rules and collective lockdowns – it seemed that none of us would be able to emerge unscathed.

I did what I could: I informed myself, read everything there was to read about the new disease, listened to the relevant podcasts and diligently took all the recommended precautions. And I threw myself into work, partly because it was good for me, partly because I didn't have any other option. The pandemic had also led to all of my events, readings and panel discussions being cancelled. I had been looking forward to some of them, to giving the closing lecture at a psychology congress, for example, which in previous years had been given by a number of writers whom I deeply admired. To a literary festival in the South of France, which, alongside some interesting encounters, had promised lovely weather. These cancellations also meant that I was losing money. I postponed writing the texts I wanted to write and sought out commissions for articles, editorial jobs and translations, often at a lower rate than I would usually have agreed to. I was grateful that this was something that was possible for me, but I had to work harder than I ever had in my life, and I missed the kind of writing that had made me choose this profession in the first place. It all felt like a loss of meaning that I could not adequately put into words.

Whenever I wasn't working, I was following the grim news, including from countries in which I had once lived or spent a lot of time. I saw, time and again, the incompetence of politicians costing countless lives, which in turn made Germany's political response to the crisis seem, perhaps, slightly more reasonable than it actually was. I was worried about my friends in New York and London, and the occasional emails and phone calls didn't make me feel any better. I felt as if life in those place that had once been so important to me was suddenly undergoing an irreversible change.

As the cultural life in the city ground to a halt, so too did my social life. A depressing gap opened up in my daily routine. My parents and my sister called more often than usual. Friends that I hadn't spoken to in years called briefly to ask how I was doing and to tell me how they were dealing with the situation. Some people I talked to again and again on Facetime and Zoom. But I often didn't see anyone for days, sometimes weeks, not even to go for a walk, because of the legal requirements at that time and my own caution. Even my various support group meetings, which I had been going to for almost ten years now, were put on hold. Some of them moved online, which was better than nothing, but I still missed them. All of these losses still felt dramatic to me; they also entailed a loss of meaning.

But what probably weighed the heaviest on me was that I was also becoming distanced from my closest friends. They were all simply preoccupied with their own problems, which made it difficult to connect with them. Sylvia and Heiko were juggling jobs that brought them into contact with a multitude of potentially sick people every day, while attempting to plan Lilith's home-schooling after their childcare fell through. For a long time, I didn't see them at all, and they were now also taking care of the garden on their own. Marie and Olaf also struggled to combine John's home-schooling with the demands of their jobs and the complexity of their daily lives. Sometimes I went for walks with them and their new, very cute and very fluffy dog, but our conversations often seemed to ossify. The challenges of this new era stirred up a strong nesting instinct in many people. Without exception, every friend of mine who was in a relationship seemed to be more focused on their family life. The time we had spent together before the pandemic, all of the things that we had done together as a matter of course, receded into the background with alarming speed. Sometimes I felt as if they had never happened at all. For most people, the pandemic made the world seem smaller. But if you lived alone, this global contraction meant the almost complete disappearance of any kind of closeness to other people. In addition, many of the conversations that I was still having with my friends were generally focused on the problems they were having in their respective relationships and families, which automatically seemed to have a greater weight than the supposedly manageable problems of my life alone. My reservoir of compassion kept dwindling. Sometimes I could hardly bear to listen to these people, who were so important to me, tell me about the hardships they were going through, how deeply they were suffering under the restrictions of the pandemic and the fear that was manifest everywhere. Or how some of them tried to see the positive in everything in a kind of compulsive act of displacement, almost congratulating themselves for standing on the balcony every now and again to applaud the country's poorly paid nursing staff for the dangerous work they were doing, despite the fact that they didn't have any choice about doing that work in the first place.

Of course, I also had many conversations and virtual encounters filled with intimacy and mutual understanding. But, during this period, I often felt pushed into the role of the patiently listening, nodding therapist. I like to listen and I also believe that you have to be generous and patient especially with the people who are close to you. When we are going through difficult times, we instinctively focus on ourselves and our ability to participate in other people's lives inevitably diminishes. We all do it, all the time. I recognized it all too well from my own behaviour. Under normal circumstances, it eventually balances out, we rarely all feel bad at the same time. But when everyone is afraid, when everyone suffers in parallel from the same unpredictable challenges, this balance is lost. During many of these conversations, I felt myself collapsing in on myself.

Day by day, I closed myself off more and more and threw myself deeper into my work. I felt increasingly lonely. And as per Frieda Fromm-Reichmann's observations, I couldn't really communicate that. When I did manage to express this feeling, I often felt an involuntary defensiveness from the person I was talking to. With some people, I felt an impatient hope that they would not have to talk about it; others seemed fundamentally unwilling or unable to understand what I was saying. At some point, a self-reinforcing dynamic of fear set in: the lonelier I felt, the less I could talk about it. And the less I talked about it, the lonelier I felt. Fear and isolation stop the conversation, lead only to speechlessness. And nothing is lonelier than the loneliness of not being seen, of not being known. Nothing feels like a greater loss of meaning than the silence it causes.

MOST PEOPLE WHO LOOK BACK on periods of loneliness share the feeling that, at that time, they were 'not themselves'. For many of us, Robert Weiss noted, our lonely self is an aberration of our real self. We are far more tense, more restless and much less able to concentrate than we could have ever imagined.[10] Periods of loneliness can incubate other problems, too, can make once-latent predispositions manifest, cause cyclical psychological problems to erupt again. Something similar happened to me. I was no longer 'myself'. I increasingly understood my predicament in that same light that we collectively see lonely people in: I had the feeling that I was to blame for my situation, that I had failed at something and that, somehow, I deserved everything I was going through.

After a while, I began to notice that it was becoming increasingly difficult for me to leave the house. Going shopping, a walk in the park, even, suddenly required extensive preparations. Often, I would be on the street before I realized that I had to go back upstairs having forgotten my wallet or having failed to shut the skylight in the corridor. And if I didn't go back upstairs, I felt like I had to pay the price. One time, I returned, shopping bags in hand, to a smoke-filled apartment and screaming smoke detectors. I had left the stove on with my little Bialetti espresso machine on top. Eventually I almost completely avoided leaving my flat.

There were days when I barely noticed how lonely I felt. On other days, the feeling overwhelmed me. I had to remind myself that it made sense to keep going about my daily routine. Whenever I read something about how much time most people had now, how they were using the pandemic to find themselves again, to rethink their own lives, to exercise more or learn new languages, I felt a certain envy, sometimes even a quiet rage. I had become so sensitive and fragile that anything could upset me, anything could shake me.

'Loneliness obfuscates,' writes the neurologist Giovanni Frazzetto in his book *Together, Closer*. If it persists, 'it becomes a deceiving filter through which we see ourselves, others, and the world.' It makes us more vulnerable to rejection, increases our insecurity in social situations and makes us see danger even where there is none.[11] In retrospect, I can see that my own vision was obfuscated. I had the feeling that I was immensely needy and that this neediness only made the people whom I came into contact with shy away from me. I reacted to other people with an excessive sensitivity. If someone wrote me a nice message, it was all I could do to stop myself from responding with an overflowing abundance of heart and kiss emojis. If someone cancelled a walk we had planned together or was distracted during a conversation, I felt offended to an almost absurd degree, taking it as a clear sign that they didn't like me anymore. Sometimes I was afraid that I had been seized by some sort of mild social paranoia. Part of me felt ridiculous about all of this, another part of me wanted to isolate myself even more, ignore anyone who was trying to get in touch and wait until all of these strange feelings had dissipated and I felt like myself again.

IN THE LAST ESSAY she wrote before her death, the psychoanalyst Melanie Klein also dealt with loneliness. She defined it as a 'yearning', a 'a ubiquitous yearning for an unattainable perfect internal state', a state of inner peace that comes from fully understanding other people and being fully understood by other people. The key issue for Klein was that this state is not attainable for any of us. On our journey through our lives, we all yearn to be accompanied emotionally and psychologically; we yearn to be seen, to be recognized and understood. But other people, Klein says, are never able or willing to do this to the extent that we desire it. Nor are we ourselves. This is a fundamental condition of life.[12]

Klein attributed this to the anxiety experienced by the young child as it forms its understanding of the world and begins learning how to speak. Learning to speak is a deeply ambivalent experience, she believed. Moments of happiness and relief are accompanied by the realization that language will never be able to replace that preverbal mutual understanding that once existed between infant and caregiver. The longing for understanding without words will never leave children, even when they are adults, nor will the disillusionment that this yearning is unfulfillable.

In essence, Klein provided a psychoanalytical explanation for the often-unbearable loss of meaning that accompanies experiences of loneliness. We are all on our own, thrown into the world. Normally our psyche protects us from having any kind of insight into this unavoidable, existential loneliness; normally we live in the fantasy that we are, indeed, understood and that other people really understand us. The pain of loneliness lies in the collapse of this fantasy, in the failure of the fiction that we are not alone in this world, in the fact that, in the light of this failure, we realize that it is nothing but a fiction.

INEVITABLY, LONELINESS IS a feeling that will catch up with each and every one of us, no matter how many friendships we maintain, no matter whether we are in a relationship or not. It envelops us, sooner or later, when we experience great upheavals in our lives, when we are struck by illness, when relationships end, when people we love die. Or during a pandemic. Perhaps it is natural that, in periods in which 'normality' is crumbling away, the self-deceptive strategies that usually help us through life no longer function. How could they, given the daily tidal wave of sickness and death, given the danger that awaited us every day outside our own front doors? Perhaps the end of normality that so many people talked about, and which so many of us felt, also meant exactly that: a proliferation of speechlessness. A failure of the fictions on which our lives together had been based. A loss of meaning that seemed unstoppable, which seemed, at first, to call everything into question, at least for a while.

Ambiguous Losses

It might have been the loneliness I felt, which I sometimes coped with better, sometimes worse; it might have been the fears about getting ill myself and the worries about the health of the people who were important to me; it might have been the people who, with a deep and often politically fuelled contempt for others, disregarded all the precautionary measures, stoking the pandemic – whatever the cause, the feeling that I was living in a prolonged state of emergency wouldn't leave me for a long time. I had the impression that I had stumbled into something interminably provisional, that I was going through life with my breath held.

If I had to name the characteristic that best defined my life during the pandemic, it was this curious collapsing of time. Everything that had structured my year had fallen away – the trips, the birthday celebrations of my friends, family and godchildren, the summer excursions to the lakes in the countryside around Berlin, the resumption of my cultural life as autumn began. Everything that happened today could also happen tomorrow, could have happened in the weeks and months before. Time seemed to have folded in on itself.

After the first few months of being alone, I had got into the habit of going for a walk for a few hours every day. Through the Hasenheide, the large park near my flat, across Tempelhofer Feld.

No matter what the weather, no matter how much work I had to do. These long walks were a ritual to end my working days or, if I wasn't able to work, to start my morning. They gave me a chance to meet people and feel a semblance of reality in a world that no longer felt real. They differed from the walks I had previously taken in their regularity and length. I resolved to walk at least ten kilometres every day. This was an appointment I made with myself, a conscious attempt to protect my mental health.

As the seasons progressed, I often couldn't say for sure which day, week or even month it was. Somewhere along the line, I stopped noticing how nature was changing around me. It was as if my life had been packed in cotton wool, as if I was stuck in a dense fog that only parted at certain moments to reveal what was actually happening to and around me. One day I noticed that the summer heat had dried everything out, turned the grass yellow and wilted the birch trees. At some later moment in time, I suddenly registered that the drops on my mackintosh felt cooler than usual and that autumn was on its way. At some point I seemed to wake up on one of those walks to find that the leaves on most of the trees had turned and the first crowns were bare.

THE ANTHROPOLOGIST Victor Turner has described this experience of time collapsing in on itself as a phenomenon of liminality, an extended threshold state. He was building on the theory of rites of passage that his colleague Arnold van Gennep had developed. Van Gennep had observed that we enter new stages of life, shed old identities and assume new social roles by way of collective rituals – in Western societies, these might be baptisms, confirmations, marriages or funerals. Turner sought to illuminate the threshold state inherent in these rites of passage; that is to say, what happens between the end of one life stage and the beginning of the next. He described this in-between state as 'a moment in and out of time', a time of 'indeterminacy' and 'ambiguity' in which we slip through the web of classifications of the world that we have, until then, known.[1]

The pandemic felt like precisely this kind of prolonged threshold state, like a time outside of regular time in which many of the old rules and norms no longer seemed to apply. In some ways it is difficult to endure periods of liminality, not least because one does not know what will come after them. They can bring back ghosts that have long been banished, make you feel trapped, make you feel like you are stuck and unable to move on. But they also represent an opportunity. They allow one to take a look at oneself, one's life and the world around one with a certain distance, from a new perspective, and to think about things one has not wanted to or not been able to think about for a long time. For me, this was my life alone.

What was often difficult for me as a single person in a world largely made up of couples and families was dealing with the lack of stability of the many friendships in my life and with the extended vicissitudes to which these friendships were subject. I became particularly aware of this during the pandemic and as I noticed the deepening nesting instincts that it triggered. I had always believed that my friends represented an unconventional, extended family for me. Isolated, I lost my faith in this belief. The change in my relationships solidified and created a new reality of its own over the course of those shapeless weeks and months that seemed to bleed into one another. A temporary distance became something that felt like a permanent distance, a distance that I only in theory understood would end one day. Ultimately, the liminality of the pandemic brought up a familiar question for me that I had previously faced under different auspices: is the model of a life of friendship limited to only one phase of life? To the phase of youth and young adulthood? Was I just too old to lead a life based on friendships?

FOR YOUNG ADULTS, friendships have, of course, a particular importance. They provide support and orientation in a bewildering world and are part and parcel of the openness that is so characteristic of this phase of life. It is no coincidence that these friendships in young adulthood have been so emphatically celebrated in popular culture for decades, and it comes as no surprise that they continue to exert a strong pull on us later in life. For a long time, they have also determined my feeling about my life, and they determine how most twenty- and thirty-year-olds I know feel about their lives.

Perhaps most prominently, the American sitcom *Friends* spelled out this phenomenon on a global scale between 1994 and 2004. It is still one of the best-known and most-watched TV series in the world, and each generation of adolescents seems to discover it anew. The series about six friends in a largely fictional New York succeeded in redefining what life could be like in that phase between youth and adulthood, a phase in which platonic friendships not only determine everyday life, but also compensate structurally for the lack of a sustained romantic relationship and a stable professional career. The secret to the series is that it enacts a sense of belonging, investing friendships with a sense of security and stability that they, by definition, do not possess. This sense of belonging is transmitted to viewers, forming their experience of watching the show. In a way, Rachel, Ross, Monica, Joey, Phoebe and Chandler also become the friends of the people who followed their fictional lives on a weekly basis.

In a flood of representations of friendships in the media, this series stood out because there was a flash of something real in its fictionality. I and many other people felt the same way about any number of other TV series based around friendships, from *Seinfeld* and *Sex and the City* to *How I Met Your Mother* and *The Big Bang Theory*. The fact that these series found such a large audience is not only to do with their highly relatable, albeit mostly aspirational fantasies of a successful life. It's also because, despite all their pathos and kitsch, these shows express an idea of friendship that audiences recognize or want to recognize from their own lives.

But the crux of all of these series, that which they are always building up to, is easily overlooked. They all without exception end with their protagonists finding partners, starting families and building lives in which their previously celebrated friendships play only a secondary role or no role at all. In the end, though, the codes and rules of friendship upheld during the series no longer apply when the heroes and heroines have arrived in the safe haven of traditional romantic relationships. Their friendships, despite numerous oaths of fidelity, seem to be upheld primarily in service of one thing: preparation for a successful marriage or marriage-like relationship. These friendships play the role of a buffer to make romantic setbacks more bearable, a kind of emotional insurance that, at some point in time, is no longer needed.

I believe that many people, in their own lives, are confronted with a similar conundrum. Despite all the experiments one gets involved in during one's extended youth, one is ultimately preparing oneself for life as an 'adult' member of society, and specifically for having a relationship and starting a family. If one were to be very blunt, one could say that friendship is thus reduced to a time of transition, that it is ascribed the function of a threshold state that ends when one successfully integrates into traditional forms of cohabitation.

FRIENDSHIPS CHANGE WHEN you or your friend enters a romantic relationship. I have experienced this many times. Friendships in which you once called each other for help at eleven at night, in which you shared the most intimate details, are, at the start of a new relationship, often put on hold completely. Until they become friendships in which you are only sporadically in touch and, when you are, you find that you have little to say to each other.

Sooner or later, an attempt is usually made to integrate your friends into your new life, which is now centred on your relationship and your new family. Whether and how this works depends on, among other things, the partner of the person you are friends with. Sometimes you get on well with them, but sometimes new partners perceive relationships from their partner's previous lives as a threat, sparking off feelings of jealousy. Sometimes you are jealous yourself or don't like someone's new partners; you might have the impression that they are not good for the person you were once so close to.

This is especially hard when you are the one who is left behind and who stays alone. At some point, you have to come to terms with being second or third in line for people you thought would always play a very important role in your life. Most of the time, you can't blame anyone for this demotion because you know that similar shifts would occur if you were in their shoes. Because it is part of the character of every friendship that they change over the course of one's life.

It is, still, however, hard to take. You feel abandoned, and you are confronted with a void that you don't at first know how to fill. The person who was once so close to you is still there, but at the same time they are absent. In some respects, this is tantamount to an 'ambiguous loss'. This concept goes back to the psychologist Pauline Boss and describes a loss in which what has been lost remains unclear. Some of the best-known and best-researched examples of ambiguous loss include mourning people with dementia who are still alive but whose personality is gradually disappearing, or mourning someone who is missing presumed dead. Ambiguous losses are characterized by a lack of information, a paradox of presence and absence, a 'both / and', an ambivalence that causes the grieving process to stall or fail altogether. Finding ways to cope with this new situation, being able to make essential decisions about one's new life, to move on and start again – this ambivalence makes these things extremely difficult. According to Boss, ambiguous loss is accompanied by its own form of trauma.[2]

THE IDEA OF THE COUPLE shapes our lives; it also determines the way in which we see the world. We describe people as 'unattached', 'single' or 'divorced' – all these designations are defined in opposition to an assumed standard – that of the couple and the nuclear family.[3] One can certainly question, however, whether this assumed standard model actually makes any sense. The British artist and essayist Hannah Black does exactly that in her radically perceptive essay 'The Love of Others', in which she describes the couple as the 'most reductive, exclusionary and precarious imaginable method of meeting the probably universal need to feel close to and recognized by others'.[4] In its heterosexual form, Black goes so far as to call life in a couple a 'patriarchal horror movie'. She cites the concomitant emotional and psychological labour, the financial dependence and domestic violence that women experience in these relationships. Queer couples, she attests, recreate 'this structure of violence, domination and emotional paucity'. And yet, the power of the idea of the couple remains undimmed; it has displaced every other model for living, including a life lived through friendships.

On my darker days, I find it hard not to agree with Black's striking logic. Dark days when I also think back to a conversation I had with a friend that struck a similar chord. We had gone to see an exhibition of queer photographers from the 1970s and 1980s in SoHo. One of the artists we both admired most, Peter Hujar, was among their number; I had been moved by his black-and-white photographs for many years. The day before the visit to the gallery, I had gone to see my ex-boyfriend in our former flat in Park Slope, where he still lived. He was now married to a lovely man several years my junior and, with the help of a surrogate, was becoming a father, creating a kind of model gay family. Of the artists on show in the exhibition, none had led happy romantic lives, not even Hujar. Most of them had often struggled with great loneliness and had died far too young.

I asked my friend if she thought that friendship could genuinely be a model for life, a model that could compensate for or replace the absence of a romantic relationship. I realized that, simply in the hopeful way I had posed the question, I was already succumbing to a degree of fantasy, a kind of projected wish fulfilment. Hanya just shook her head. In the end, she said, you are always alone when you are single. In the end, everyone, including your best friends, will find a relationship and will hardly have any time for you. I refuse to believe that, I said. I'm not sure whether my response would be the same today.

BUT HOW MUCH did I really want to share my life with someone again? Romantic relationships can feel like a safe haven, mediocre and beautiful, but they can also spiral out of control, be defined by a dissolving of one's boundaries, and that too can be beautiful in its own way. I had experienced both and, on some days, both felt like a better version of life than the one I was leading. And yet, at some point, I stopped longing for a romantic relationship. Perhaps it had become too painful for me, perhaps a kind of sustained hopelessness had set in. A hopelessness masquerading as pragmatism, a reasonable view of the world and of one's place in it. Of course, there were still days when my longing and my desire caught up with me; and it was not as if my life, over the past few years, had been completely devoid of physical intimacy. Irregularly, I went on dates, met a man for dinner, a coffee, a museum visit. Sometimes I had the feeling that these men recognized a need in me that I kept so hidden from myself that it shocked me to see it reflected back to me in their faces. Sometimes, though, I slept with them. But even if we slept together again after that, I never felt any sense of intimacy, and I had the impression that I was the root cause of this. That I was denying myself something.

During the pandemic, of course, these kinds of encounters did not take place. And, actually, I was glad of it. It would have been too difficult to fight the inner belief that underlay each of these encounters and which, at that time, I felt particularly strongly. A belief that had endured many years of psychoanalysis, therapy and self-help groups, that had shifted, metamorphosed and undergone occasional hiatuses, but had never completely disappeared: the belief that I could not really be loved, was not, in any real sense, lovable. That I and my body were not suitable for being met with desire, not suitable for somebody to project their romantic and sexual fantasies upon. And that life with me was too challenging anyway, that my psychological problems were too severe to regularly inflict on another person in an unfiltered way.

Of course, I knew that this belief was, to some extent, irrational. I had reflected on its causes, had learned, when possible, to avoid it, to confront it, to live with it. But that didn't change the fact that it kept recurring and remained part of the basic grammar of the way I perceived myself. Carrying this belief around with me inevitably meant denying myself what I longed for. How are you supposed to change such deep-seated assumptions about yourself when they feel like incontrovertible truths? It's easier just to set that longing aside, at least for a while.

IN SOME WAYS, when you live alone, your whole life can be described as an 'ambiguous loss', in the way that Pauline Boss defines it. One mourns the loss of a partner one no longer has, or never has had. One vacillates between optimism, sadness and suppression and tries, when things get very bad, to divorce oneself, altogether, from the concept of a life lived together. A concept you have to mourn, even though you feel you shouldn't have to.

The older you get, the bigger the conglomeration of these ambiguous losses becomes. They show up in the most surprising moments. Most of the time you deal with them in a practised way, focusing on the aspects of everyday life that work well, the things you can be happy about. Then one day you go for a walk in Hasenheide park, the sun hasn't shone for a long time, the news is once again full of overwhelming horrors and, suddenly, there is a father who is teaching his little two-year-old daughter to play football. She is surprisingly skilled, quickly learning to knock the ball forward with one little leg, running after it and then jockeying it again with the other little leg, all the while applying the greatest concentration. And if you're not careful, tears are going to fill your eyes, outside, in the middle of the park, because once you would have liked to have become just this kind of father, because once you had believed that you would become one.

The most difficult thing about the ambiguous losses of a life alone is not how you grieve the absent relationship. The most difficult thing is saying goodbye to all the notions you had for your life, the many fantasies – the fulfilment of which you once took for granted. You grieve a model of life that you not only watch being lived out everywhere around you, but one that you too have internalized. You have to learn to detach yourself from the idea that you will one day start a family, have children and watch them grow up, that at some point you will be able to look back on a life lived together and say: you know, in the end it was pretty good.

Sooner or later, inevitably, the fantasies required for any form of romance, any form of togetherness, begin to slip away. In her illuminating book *Desire / Love*, Lauren Berlant examines how much we do, in fact, need the power of our imagination in order to love. For her, love is above all a dream in which our desire is reciprocated, a dream fuelled by our sexual desires, by cultural ideas and by the psychological power of social institutions like marriage. It is only because of this dream plan, Berlant argues, that we are able to bear the ambivalence of the person we love and to endure the fundamental insecurity of our relationships. 'Whether viewed psychoanalytically, institutionally, or ideologically,' she writes, 'love is deemed always an outcome of fantasy.'[5] It is our imagination alone that gifts us the magic of devotion.

For the longest time, I did not lack fantasies about intimacy and love; the opposite, in fact: I had an excess. But the accumulation of those ambiguous losses, the notions of life that I had to say goodbye to, meant that I ran out of the strength to sustain these much-needed fantasies. Rather than continue to live with them, I let go. Somehow, it seemed to make more sense.

IN HIS BOOK *Liquid Love,* the sociologist Zygmunt Bauman described romantic relationships as the most frequent, most intensely experienced and most disturbing embodiment of ambivalence in the fluid life of modernity. They vacillate between 'a sweet dream and a nightmare', he writes, and for this very reason take centre stage in our therapeutic society.[6] It is worth adding that this is not only true for people in relationships. For those of us who do not have romantic relationships, they are often simultaneously 'a dream and a nightmare'. It may, in fact, be the case that, for us, this dissonance is even more pronounced.

Some years ago, I spent a few months in London, where I found myself dealing with a depression that the end of a difficult relationship had plunged me into. A conversation I had had about it led a friend to take me to a support group meeting called 'Sex and Love Addicts Anonymous'. I had no idea why Tom thought that this group could help me. I was aware of the feeling that sex and love had an addictive side, particularly from those years in which I had partied a lot, drank a lot and took a lot of drugs. But I was sure that these were things that were no longer relevant to the life I was now leading. I had grown up so much since then, had become so sensible. But, to my surprise, these group meetings were a revelation. Although, in many ways, my life appeared to be quite different to that of many of the other people there, I found that I could relate to them incredibly well.

One of the topics discussed in the group that particularly fascin-ated me was the concept of 'sexual and emotional anorexia'.[7] I felt like I immediately understood what it meant. Other people felt the same way, whether they had just come directly from their third visit to a sex club that week, ashamed, or, for ten years, had been grieving their relationship with an ex-boyfriend, without trying to embark on a new relationship. In the group's recommended literature, I read that sexual and emotional anorexia is characterized by the uncon-scious maintenance of a state of emotional starvation and often, without knowing it, the development of a series of avoidance strat-egies. When one senses that something like intimacy with a person might be possible, one rejects that person, based on past experiences, because one cannot stand one's own vulnerability. In many cases, there is a dynamic of excess and renunciation, sexual excess and then abstinence, complete loss of control and then total control. It is a dynamic that is hard to identify in oneself. A dynamic that leads to one not getting what one wants and needs most: real intimacy.

Emotional and sexual anorexia is not a psychiatric diagnosis. I have only ever come across the concept in these meetings and their recommended reading, and in a couple of essays in American psychology journals. A few years later, when I told a therapist about this self-diagnosis, he could do little with it. Nevertheless, it was a concept that I found enormously helpful. Here, for the first time, I had found a convincing explanation for those aspects of my life that I had struggled to understand.

I clung to this idea for a long time. I explained it to friends and reminded myself of it whenever someone tried to kiss me after a date or even just flirt with me, whenever I wandered the streets of Berlin, wanting to feel as invisible as possible. These days, though, I'm not so sure whether it does, in fact, describe me and my feelings that well. I wonder, whether, over the years, this notion that was once so helpful to me hasn't in fact become something that it was never meant to be: a variation of that old refrain – the one that says that love is for other people, not for me. The manifest proof that I am too damaged to put myself out there for another person, too damaged to be capable of true intimacy. The proof that I, this conglomeration of psychiatric symptoms, am doing the right thing by remaining alone. The ultimate proof that I am unlovable.

IN THOSE MONTHS in London, attending the group's meetings and dealing with my emotional anorexia, I had also taken up smoking again. Now, five years later, at the height of the pandemic, I stopped. Maybe it had to do with my fear of the virus and the pneumonia it could cause. But maybe the long daily walks had also set something in motion. And maybe I needed to take back at least a little control during a period in which nothing seemed controllable.

I knew that the cessation of social life during the pandemic, that liminal time, had caused me to lose my footing. Not least because I was missing all the well-rehearsed and well-loved rituals of my everyday life I shared with my friends. All of us look for support in the rituals of a shared everyday life. As the sociologist Janosch Schobin explains, it is its order and its recurring rhythms that create one of our most important fictions: the sense that things will always go on as they have done, the feeling of 'infinity' that we associate with the idea of a secure future. In other words, it is the everydayness of our relationships that give us a sense of dependability and stability; in some sense, it has the power to banish or at least diminish 'the mortal's fear of death'.[8]

During those months, this fear was difficult for me to brush off. It was probably for this reason that I also began to reshape and renew my daily routine, which had largely crumbled. In addition to my morning or afternoon walks, I began, in the evenings, to watch some of the TV series I mentioned above, centred around circles of friends. I had watched most of them at some time or other and, at its most basic, my reunion with these old acquaintances was a comfort to me. There was something soothing about it and, though I couldn't quite put my finger on exactly why, it felt like a welcome substitute for a real everyday life.

I also started knitting almost every evening. It was the ideal accompaniment to the undemanding TV series I was watching and allowed me to do something useful as I sat there. For several years I had been looking for pastimes that had nothing to do with my work. Besides French classes, I took a painting course and, for a summer, spent every Friday afternoon in the Botanical Garden learning how to paint China asters, dahlias and sunflowers. I learned to crochet and spent a winter making a large multi-coloured blanket in a Celtic knot pattern. Activities like these relaxed me, even if, at first, they could feel a little silly. Over the years they had become a means of helping me through the turbulence of life, allowing me to calm down for a moment.

There was also something deeply meditative about knitting every evening. It seemed to connect me very directly to the world, to bind me more tightly to the presence of my life. I knitted some wristbands and socks for myself and a few friends. And, as my skills improved, I made mittens, hats, jumpers and cardigans in the brightest neon colours I could find for the little kids in my circle of friends and acquaintances.

Knitting is remarkably complex. It takes a lot more practice than you might at first think, and it is deeply satisfying when you notice yourself becoming more skilled, the stitches becoming more even and the garments more beautiful. Eventually, you even learn techniques to realize details like buttonholes that won't wear out, shoulders that fit properly or cuffs that are tight but not too tight. But at the same time, you constantly face new, dizzying obstacles. When you first hold a set of five thin sock knitting needles for the first time you doubt all principles of logic and geometry. Not to mention when it comes to the more complicated cable knits, Arans, brioche and lace patterns you hope to one day master, or to multicoloured jacquard and intarsia knitting.

Perhaps there is something so reassuring about knitting because it connects you to the collective knowledge of past generations. To our mothers, grandmothers and great-grandmothers and all their collective hopes, loves and disappointments. To the Mongolian nomads who made warm clothes from the wool of their yaks, the men from the Scottish Highlands who wove their sheep's wool, the famous *tricoteuses* who knitted the iconic *bonnets rouges* during the French Revolution. Like all of these people, you transform a ball of wool into something you can wear, transfer the chaos of life into a new order. You don't just make a garment, you make meaning. And unlike in real life, you have the chance to repair dropped stitches and other mistakes, or even unravel the knitted piece altogether, wind the yarn back up into a ball and make something completely new out of it. Knitting is the perfect pastime when the world gets colder, the perfect pastime for a pandemic. You take your loneliness and make something beautiful out of it.[9]

Victor Turner described these liminal experiences – such as the one we experienced during the pandemic – as 'a time and place of withdrawal from normal modes of social action', a phase in which we also review and reconsider the 'central values and axioms' of our lives and culture.[10] For him, this state was always associated with a kind of meditative reflection, a thinking about oneself and the world, a 'juggling with the factors of existence', as he called it.[11] The ethnologist recognized in liminality a universal category of human experience, one of the central ingredients of the drama and mystery of being alive.

Looking back on those months that, for me, seemed to flow into each other, I realize that those 'factors of existence' I was juggling with were different from the factors that I had imagined at the time. Of course, the news determined my everyday life. Of course, I missed those people who were close to me, missed them a lot. But I also began to live with my loneliness in a new way, to face all those ambiguous losses that I had not wanted to think about for so long.

How can one mourn losses that are ambiguous? How can we say goodbye to what we ourselves find difficult just to name? We want grief to be finite, to have, at some point, an end, but in truth, we grieve, continue our lives, grieve again, grieve anew, continue to grieve, and sometimes losses can be so ambiguous that our grief has no end.[12] I began working on my grief by admitting to myself that I felt lost, that my attempts at finding an explanation for my being alone had reached their limit, had, in a way, failed. Perhaps this would be a first step towards finding myself again.

Little by little, I tried to consciously say goodbye to the idea that one day I would find that person with whom I wanted to grow old and start a family. I also tried to say goodbye to the idea that my friends could be something like a substitute for the romantic relationship I didn't have, that my friendships would save me from being alone. Sometimes we hold on to something with all our might and cannot let it go because we have become so used to the pain of holding on, because we are used to things hurting. Perhaps this was the case for me too. Slowly I began to unravel the knitting of my life, to make something new out of its threads. I just didn't yet know what.

Days in Famara

A few days into the New Year, an acquaintance of mine was found dead in his flat. I heard about it through a mutual friend. Peter had been my age. He had run a successful practice as a psychotherapist, was friends with everyone and was able to quickly win people over with his wit and his charm. From the outside, he led a wonderful life. Over the previous few months, I had largely ignored his calls. Like many other gay men I knew, his initially carefree partygoing had turned into a severe addiction over the years, with all of its dramatic consequences. I had met him when he first sought help. After a year of living without crystal meth, GHB and MDMA, the drugs that, among other things, helped him to overcome his sexual inhibitions, he fell into a cycle of relapses and periods of hope. The people in his life were heartbroken. He died of an overdose. The man he had been with that night had fled the scene. It was impossible to say whether Peter's death was an accident, whether he had been killed or whether he had wanted to take his own life.

The news of his death came at a time when, despite occasional glimmers of hope, a sense of desolation kept catching up with me. The pandemic had been going on for almost a year by then. After some careful preparations, I had spent Christmas with Marie, Olaf and John again, but had seen few people before or after, and when I did, it was only for a walk. I had stopped using public transport. The city's museums, cinemas, operas, theatres and concert halls had been closed for so long that I had almost forgotten that they were ever there. Much of what had once held my life together had simply ceased to exist. I hadn't touched a person in almost a year, hadn't hugged anyone except for rare, spontaneous slip-ups.

To add to this, the number of cases worldwide had reached a new high after the holidays, and more easily transmissible and danger-ous virus variants had been discovered in Great Britain and South Africa, and it seemed likely that they were going to quickly spread across the globe. I had the impression that, all around me, people were dying, the parents and grandparents of friends, but also people like Peter. I wasn't the only one wondering, even, if the pandemic were to end soon, how many traumas we would all have to learn to live with over the coming years.

TRAVELLING WAS NOT FORBIDDEN, but it was certainly still being advised against in no uncertain terms. Over the previous few weeks, I had been debating back and forth with two of my best friends, David and Rafa, about whether we should go. We had planned the trip to Lanzarote in the summer, when hardly anyone really wanted to believe that the pandemic would be with us in one way or another for several years. During a long walk a few days before our flight, I asked Gabriele – a seventy-year-old friend whose counsel I almost always trusted – whether our break was really justifiable during times like these. Not really, she said, but you have to go, of course. Despite the difficulties, obstacles and risks involved. It would do me good, she said, and you had to make these kinds of exceptions. We all made them; otherwise one couldn't survive situations like this.

By the time we were approaching Famara, a village on the west coast of the island, I knew that I had made the right decision. The bright-blue evening sky arched above the volcanic fields and mountains, their colours changing from a bright rusty red to deep black. On the horizon, we could see the streaks of spray in the shifting bay. We passed palm trees, and the whole alien, moon-like landscape was dotted with little bright-green plants and shrubs that had sprouted after the rain a few days earlier. My body, still reeling from the Berlin winter, rejoiced. We had lowered the roof of the convertible. I felt the warm breeze on my face, and behind my sunglasses, my eyes tried to adjust to this new light. All three of us were on the island for the first time. We were experiencing all of this together, having an experience we had never had before. I hadn't realized how much I had missed this simple aspect of life.

EVEN THE MOST optimistic single people occasionally express just how unlikely it feels that they will ever be in a romantic relationship again. I could remember countless conversations with friends in which they expressed exactly this kind of hopelessness, expressed a feeling of being excluded from the world, from those who can love and can be loved. At the time, I never really understood them properly, always told them how distorted their view of their own situation was. But now that the tide had turned, now that most of these friends were in relationships and it was I who was alone, I thought, as I said, differently about these things.

I did, however, wonder if hopelessness was really the right word for what I was feeling. Somehow it felt more contained and at the same time more desperate. In his book *Mourning Diary*, Roland Barthes introduces the term *acedia* in this context, a notion that really resonated with me. The word, which originates from early Christianity, was used by Barthes to mean an 'apprehensiveness', a 'bitterness or a 'hardness of the heart'. For Barthes, *acedia* describes not the loss of one's faith in love, but the loss of one's interest in it.[1] He defines it as 'unexcitability', the 'inability to love', and adds the following to describe this state more precisely: 'Anguished because I don't know how to restore generosity to my life – or love. How to love?'[2] That was exactly what I felt. Exactly the question I was asking myself.

Barthes was not alone in reflecting on the effects of this kind of romantic hopelessness in his life. The psychologist Walt Odets, who has run a psychotherapeutic practice in Berkeley for many decades, has also returned time and again to very similar reflections. In his book *Out of the Shadows*, he describes how these kinds of feelings are particularly prevalent among gay men.[3] I think this is true for many queer people, be they lesbian, gay, bisexual or transgender. For many of us, what we were warned about as teenagers, often even with the best of intentions, seems to have come to pass: that our otherness would ensure a life spent alone, without love.

THE FIRST TIME I felt this kind of hopelessness, this *acedia*, was in the early 1990s. I was fourteen and in love with a boy from another class in my year. He was handsome, had long blond hair and exuded a confidence that seemed to say that he had never questioned himself, his body or his sexuality. As far as I knew, I was the only gay boy at the small provincial high school in Mecklenburg where, of course, the gay liberation movement had not yet made its presence known.

If there were other gay boys, they were better at hiding it than I was. And it was a time to hide. The AIDS epidemic dominated the news and was wiping out an entire generation of gay men. To be gay was to spread the most stigmatized disease that had ever existed. The whole world seemed to hate us, to be waiting for us to die. There was never any question that sexual experimentation or even anything that might come close to a whirlwind romance was possible for me. Later, perhaps, at a time that seemed very far away, but not in that moment.

Sometimes you hide yourself away so well that you don't know who you are any more. It has an enduring effect, this going into hiding at a time of life during which, without being aware of it, you learn almost everything about yourself. During which you learn who you are, who you could be, who you are allowed to be. Many years later, when I was living in Park Slope with my partner, going to the farmer's market on Saturdays, shopping for the week and thinking about where we would go dancing that evening, I actually thought that the hide-and-seek of my youth had nothing to do with me anymore. I remember a session with Ona, the psychoanalyst I was seeing at the time. I had been seeing her regularly for six months because, no matter what I did, my depression always caught up with me eventually and sometimes I didn't even know why I was alive anymore. We had circled some problematic areas, we had talked about my eating disorder, about why I drank so much, had such a problematic relationship with my body, how much sexual validation I needed, why I had cheated on my partner despite resolving not to do so. Sooner or later, we almost always got stuck. At one point she asked me if I was ashamed of being gay. With a vehemence that surprised me, I said no. For years, I had been completely open about my sexuality. I lived with a man, in a city where that was not unusual. Why should I feel anything like shame? Ona said nothing and only raised her eyebrows at the vehemence of my reaction.

I ENJOYED TRAVELLING with Rafa and David. We had been going on trips together for a few years now. We celebrated my fortieth birthday in Paris, went to see the Venice Biennale and wandered around Madrid searching for a celebrated Peruvian restaurant. Over the years, first Rafa had found a partner and now David was in a relationship too, and it seemed like it was going to be long term. I liked their boyfriends. And despite their changed circumstances, the three of us still enjoyed travelling together.

Rafa is ten years younger and David fifteen years older than I am. In a way, we belong to three different generations of gay men. David comes from the generation that was fully exposed to the deadly horror of the AIDS epidemic. I come from a generation that grew up with the news and knowledge of these horrors, but came of age at a time when the disease was increasingly contained. And Rafa is from a generation for whom none of these things seemed to matter much anymore, and who take for granted many of the formerly unimaginable rights and freedoms that queer people have today. Each of our generations has to deal with different traumas of shame. Each has built a life around them their own way.

SHAME, ESPECIALLY IN THE LIVES of queer people, is more than just a feeling. Eve Kosofsky Sedgwick has described it as a kind of free radical that can attach itself to almost anything, changing its meaning. Whether it's our understanding of our own bodies, certain behaviours, our feelings: queer shame, she writes, affects all of our relationships and determines how we understand ourselves.[4]

In his book *The Velvet Rage*, the psychologist Alan Downs explored the extent of this shame. Using the example of gay men, Downs shows how many queer people learn during childhood and adolescence that their desire is less 'plausible' or 'natural' than that of heterosexual people. He describes the resulting shame as something that becomes an internal organizing principle over the course of one's life, something that one always has to fight against and compensate for. What starts out as just a feeling, he believes, burrows deep into our psyches, becoming something more unfathomable, a more deeply felt, more rigid belief that there is not only something fundamentally wrong with us, but that, if we want to survive, we have to work to make something of ourselves that can be loved.[5]

Queer shame is not only the product of a psychological dynamic, it is also socially institutionalized. As Didier Eribon elucidates in his book *Insult and the Making of the Gay Self*, this happens, for instance, through the many stigmatizing insults and derogatory categorizations that queer people experience and which, in a sense, assign them their places in the patriarchal society in which we live. We all grow up intuitively knowing which genders, sexualities and bodies occupy which hierarchical position in the world around us. Which relationships with the people we love are 'right' and which are 'wrong'. This knowledge is an indelible part of us. It is confirmed again and again by the majority of society. Even if we reject it, we carry it with us.[6]

These psychological dynamics and social institutionalizations of shame also have a long history. A history that, in Germany, is particularly unequivocal. The Nazi regime labelled homosexuals 'degenerate' and a threat to the 'masculine character' of the 'German national body'. Their declared aim was to eradicate homosexuality. Even 'covetous looks' were enough for criminal prosecution. Gay men were tortured, chemically castrated and subjected to medical experiments. It is estimated that up to 15,000 queer people were deported to concentration camps, where over half of them were murdered. And their persecution did not stop after the end of Nazi rule and the cessation of the Second World War. Some of them, after surviving the concentration camps, were interned again by the occupying powers.

For many decades, gay men, lesbians and trans people were not counted among the victims of National Socialism. Their rights did not count as human rights, and they were excluded from the protections offered by West Germany's new constitution, the Grundgesetz. Paragraph 175 of the German criminal code, which had made male homosexuality a punishable offence since the founding of the German Reich in 1871, was almost abolished in the Weimar Republic. But it was retained in post-war West Germany and was used in over 100,000 trials, leading to the conviction of over 50,000 gay men. From today's perspective, it is difficult to truly comprehend what the lives of those men affected by this persecution were like, although, from a historical point of view, this did not occur all that long ago. It is difficult to grasp the inner constraint and latent horror that must have been required to live in a society that rejected them, persecuted them and made them susceptible to blackmail, that forced them to suppress their natural desires and, if they engaged with them at all, to do so only in secret. It condemned them to forego a fulfilled life, to never fully living their humanity.

It was not until 1969 that homosexuality among men over the age of 21 was decriminalized in West Germany, followed in 1972 by the decriminalization of homosexuality among men over the age of eighteen. In East Germany, these same laws had been passed in 1957 and 1968, respectively. However, here too lesbians and gays were monitored, discriminated against, antagonized and persecuted as representatives of a 'bourgeois' lifestyle. It was not until 1990 that the World Health Organization removed homosexuality from its catalogue of mental illnesses. It was not until 1994, when I was sixteen, that Paragraph 175 was finally removed from the penal code in reunified Germany. It was not until 2002 that the homosexual victims of National Socialism were rehabilitated by the Bundestag, and it was not until March 2017 that the same occurred for the victims of West Germany's criminal prosecutions. Many of the men affected had been dead for years by then. It was only in October 2017 that the law in Germany changed to allow same-sex couples to marry. And only since December 2018 have Germans had the right to officially identify as non-binary.[7]

The past, as we know, is never really in the past. What once was, writes the French sociologist Pierre Bourdieu, is inscribed forever not only in our history, but in our social being, in our objects and also in our bodies. Our history still determines our patterns of thought and perception in the present day.[8] If a society treats a group of people over centuries and decades as if they were criminals, as if they were sick and worthless, it is difficult to prevent this group of people from internalizing exactly these attributions. It is almost always the case, even today, that the judgements of the white, patriarchally structured majority count more than the judgements we form about ourselves, writes Roxane Gay. We accept these judgements. According to Gay, they spread like an infection throughout our bodies. They turn into depression or addiction or some other physical manifestation of our silence.[9] All of this can feel like a form of sexualized violence, and in fact it is just that: a form of sexualized violence.

TODAY I CAN RECOGNIZE queer shame in myself. When on bad days I avoid other people, especially other gay men, on the street and walk with my head down, staring at the pavement. When I keep away from someone I find attractive, fearing that he might realize how I feel. When I'm down and start eating compulsively again. When I starve myself, count my calories, exercise obsessively. When I suddenly become so shy that I have to consciously dig down deep into myself during an important conversation or at an event before I even dare say a word.

And it is something that I recognize in other queer people too. On the street, in gay men who give other gay men surprisingly pointed, punishing looks. In queer friends who desperately cling to their classically bourgeois lives, as if this might actually help them forget the injuries that they have suffered. In older white gay men who hold misogynistic, transphobic and racist views, with the same air of 'common sense' expressed by the majority, of which they now consider themselves to be part. In gay men who recite the litany of their sexual conquests every time you meet them and cannot escape the sometimes dystopian and toxic world of certain gay communities.[10] In the gay men, lesbian women, trans women and men in the support group whose meetings I have been attending for many years, when we talk about our experiences with alcohol and drugs, about those addictions that have determined our lives for decades and with which queer people have to struggle more often than straight people. Whenever I perceive this shame, I try to counter it with the only attitude that helps: an attitude of acceptance and love. I do not always succeed.

SHAME THRIVES IN the shadows. It was only on Lanzarote that I realized that one of the problems of my long pandemic-induced solitude was that it had also forced me to be alone with my internal conversations, with all of those reproaches, recriminations and humiliations to which I had, without really noticing it, subjected myself. When you spend your days alone, there is no one to dispel these kinds of thoughts.

In Famara, I was also getting up early. I made myself a coffee, stepped from our terrace onto the beach, cup in hand. I let the cool seawater wash around my feet and watched the sun rise behind the mountains. When I got back to the house, Rafa and David were usually up too, and we started our day by eating breakfast together. Sometimes the three of us would explore the island, driving to a particularly beautiful lookout or a restaurant that we had read about. Sometimes we each went about our own business, and the highlight of the day was a trip to the supermarket. Every evening we watched a film by Pedro Almodóvar. It was our little joint project for the holiday. Fourteen films in fourteen days. I knew most of these films, loved them, even the bad ones, and could almost always remember exactly where I was when I had first seen them. Which stage of life I was at, how important they had been to me. I remembered their rich colour, their delight in drama, absurd comedy, their intrinsic understanding of the full range of human existence, the celebration of the marginal, of the many different trajectories life can take, the gay and lesbian friendships and romances, their many transgender characters, the great actresses: Carmen Maura, Rossy de Palma, Marisa Paredes and, of course, Penélope Cruz. These characters who, against all odds, savour life with a great matter-of-factness and strike one liberating blow after the other. That perpetual, grandiose emancipation from all of the patriarchal, normative rubbish of life. We started with *Broken Embraces*, a film partly set on Lanzarote. Suddenly we all held our breath; in a few of the scenes we saw Famara. On the screen we saw our beach and, behind the beach, our mountains.

It is no surprise that it was Michel Foucault, a gay philosopher, who coined the phrase 'friendship as a way of life'. In doing so, he described a kind of friendship among queer people that had not been considered in the confines of previous philosophical notions of friendship that were limited only to heterosexual white men. He was also avoiding the trap of thinking about 'homosexuality' only in terms of sexuality, thus reducing queer people's lives to the question of whom they sleep with.[11] The concept was developed further by Didier Eribon, who was bound to Foucault in precisely this kind of intense, life-long friendship that existed outside of conventional social and family institutions. Circles of friends, Eribon explains, can represent 'the centre of a gay life' for queer people, the 'gay person's psychological (and also geographical) journey moves from solitude to socialization by means of meeting places'. Friendships, according to Eribon, are the basis for the process of 'an invention, both collective and individual, of oneself'.[12] For queer people, friendships are essential for survival; only with their help are they genuinely able to discover their own identity.

In Famara, I had the feeling that I was being reminded of exactly that, of the power that friendships can have, of how they can orientate you. The days felt like an indescribable luxury because they were full of conversations. Conversations that had been going on between us for a few years now, in which David, Rafa and I exchanged thoughts and ideas with a great matter-of-factness, in which there was a mutual understanding of the queer shame that we sometimes repressed and sometimes openly expressed – the shame that each of us had learned to live with in our own way.

Having been alone for so long, it felt good to be able to talk about how I felt – about my solitude, about my sense that I was probably going to remain alone, that it felt to me as final as Barthes' *acedia*, that dryness of the heart. Of course, we had also talked about this before. Nevertheless, something shifted in me in Famara, something loosened up a little. Something that had seemed like an irrefutable truth during the loneliness of the pandemic still seemed like a truth; it just became a little less irrefutable.

THIS DID NOT MEAN that I didn't also need time by myself to work through the everyday chaos raging in my head. At the opposite end of the beach rose Famara's massif. On the very first day of our trip, recalling my experiences at Lake Lucerne, I decided to explore the hiking trails there. The next day, David and Rafa drove me to the other side of the mountain range, to Haria, an amazingly verdant town covered in palm trees, from where I set out on my hike. I couldn't convince them to join me, and they drove off to continue exploring the island by car. It was a surprisingly beautiful and challenging hike that pushed me to the very limits of my physical strength and abilities, but rewarded me with stunning views of the sea, the coast and large parts of the island. After I had passed the summit, and the path back to Famara became a little more traversable, I was overcome with recurrent waves of euphoria. I had never seen anything like that outlandishly beautiful, barren landscape. The multicoloured rock masses, the myriad lichens on the boulders of lava, the strange succulents, cacti and euphorbia; the spherical *aulaga* and yellow-flowered giant woody sow thistles, reminiscent of huge dandelions, the lizards scurrying back and forth with their curious turquoise necks. The world up there was suffused with a kind of magic. I decided to come back as often as I could. The very next day I hiked up the mountain again, this time from Famara. For the rest of our time on the island, this became my early evening ritual, timed so that I was back at our beach by sunset, ready for dinner and movies.

During these evening walks, I thought over not only the conversations we had been having, but the things I had read, sometimes many years before. These were not epiphanies. But something made me ponder new ideas and new ways of explaining my solitude and my hopelessness. I often returned to Alan Downs, the aforementioned author of *The Velvet Rage*. For Downs, it is a given that, when young queer people's lives are primarily focused on avoiding feelings of queer shame at all costs, this inevitably leads to a number of unwanted side effects. To unstable relationships, to a toxic view of one's own body and even to my feelings of hopelessness. However, Downs also believes that, sooner or later, we can realign ourselves. At some point, he believes, you bid farewell to this preliminary life built on strategies to avoid feelings of shame so that you can reconstruct it all over again. Not quickly, not abruptly or in radical strides, but slowly and with any eye on the real possibilities that are available to you. I was starting to believe this more and more. Maybe this new phase of my life was just beginning. Maybe it had never been about whether or not I was too damaged to be loved, was too unlovable, or whether I was using my emotional anorexia to shield myself from intimacy. Maybe I was simply rebuilding my life, something that, in the first instance, I could only do alone. And maybe this process had been going on for much longer than I had realized. I couldn't tell if this was really the case. Whether life really does fit into such neat schemes, fits those kinds of models so precisely. But the thought gave me something I hadn't felt for a long time: hope.

During my early evening hikes up the mountain, I rarely met other people. But on the way down, I saw the same hiker almost every time; he seemed to have a similar evening ritual to mine, setting off just a little later. He was always dressed head to toe in black hiking gear and was about my age, with a moustache and long dark hair that was already starting to show a little grey. He seemed likeable somehow. I couldn't tell if he lived on the island or, like me, was just visiting. The first few times our paths crossed, we greeted each other with just a quick '*¡Hola!*' and a nod. A few evenings later, I mentioned this man to David and Rafa, and it struck me that he had made a bigger impression on me than I had first thought. After a few more encounters, we smiled at each other when we crossed paths. He probably also wondered who I was and what I was doing on the mountain every evening. David, Rafa and I eventually started making all kinds of assumptions about him. And I discovered that a part of me was always looking out for him and was a bit disappointed if I didn't see him. But, at some point, just as our trip was coming to an end, we stopped, smiled at each other, and he asked, simply: '*¿Qué tal?*'

THE CONVERSATIONS THAT David, Rafa and I had had also touched on Peter. All three of us had known him. We had shared the hope he felt when he first sought help, tried to help him ourselves, had shared a lot of laughter with him. We had all watched his downward spiral during the last months of his life, had seen how his confidence ebbed away after each new setback. We had seen the shame and self-hatred in his face, in how he held himself, and how much he suffered from loneliness, the loneliness of addiction, the loneliness of the pandemic. We all understood how this could happen to someone; all three of us had been on a similar path at some point in our lives. We knew we had been lucky, very lucky. Lucky to still be alive.

Bodywork

People have always been lonely. They have experienced this feeling always and everywhere, and they have used all their strength to try and evade it. Loneliness is not a modern or even a contemporary phenomenon. No matter what our beliefs are about earlier eras and cultures, no matter what pastoral, religious and social idylls we project onto the past, loneliness is something that has always been recorded in philosophy and literature. In one way or another, in different culturally specific variations. The ancient Babylonian *Epic of Gilgamesh*, the origins of which go back to the early third millennium BC, deals with loneliness. It tells the story of a friendship between Gilgamesh, demigod and king of Uruk, and Enkidu, but it also focuses on Gilgamesh's grief and loneliness after the death of his friend. In ancient Greece, we find the myths of Prometheus, Oedipus and Sisyphus and how they experienced social isolation and pain in their different ways. In the Old Testament, God created Eve and thus humanity, because he understood that man should not be alone. Ovid's *Metamorphoses* gave us the myth of Narcissus, who perishes in the face of the loneliness of his permanent self-reflection and his inability to break out of his mental prison.

And, when you take a closer look, you also notice that the centuries-old literature of friendship is, ultimately, a literature of loneliness, of solitude and grief. As Jacques Derrida points out in his book *The Politics of Friendship*, these texts were written almost exclusively from a testamentary perspective. They memorialize deceased friends and in doing so reflect on what it meant for the author to be left behind.[1]

None of us can escape loneliness. It is an unavoidable, existential experience. Perhaps also a necessary one.

TOWARDS THE END of our stay on Lanzarote, I realized that I did not want to return to Berlin under any circumstances. I was shocked by the strength of this feeling. Maybe it was the company of Rafa and David, maybe it was the hiking in the mountains, the sun, the extraordinary landscape, the verdant spring, the sound of the Atlantic waves. I suddenly became aware of the weight I had been carrying around with me for the past months, the whole time, everywhere I went. I understood that I was stuck and was just about to take the first steps to getting myself out of my predicament, and that these first steps were actually having an effect. I was afraid that this process would stop again in Berlin and that I would be infected by the city's tired, dark mood, which seemed to have reached a nadir around that time.

A few weeks earlier, I had reread Roland Barthes' *Mourning Diary*, written after the death of his mother. In this slim book, what becomes palpable is the fact that being alive can sometimes feel like a problem. Like an inescapable problem for which there is no solution. I felt much the same way. I recognized the signs of an approaching depression and knew that I would not get through another one. A few years earlier, a psychiatrist had recommended that I spend my winters in the south, in the sun. The idea had always seemed absurd to me, too expensive and also impracticable because my schedule was usually full of lectures and readings. But, during the pandemic, there were no events, and those that took place were online. I talked it over with David and Rafa, scraped together all the money I had left in my account and asked Tim, my neighbour in Berlin, if he would continue emptying my mailbox and taking care of the not completely hardy patio plants that I had put in the kitchen to overwinter. Then I rented a holiday apartment in a small coastal town on Fuerteventura, the neighbouring Canary Island.

THERE WAS, OF COURSE, a paradox in me deliberately seeking solitude while struggling with feelings of loss and loneliness. But even as I stood on the deck of the ferry, breathing in the sea air and watching the island landscape of Lanzarote slowly dissipate on the horizon, I had the feeling that maybe this wasn't as absurd as it had at first seemed. And once I had moved into my little apartment, unpacked my suitcase, put my hiking boots by the door and my laptop on the dining table, I knew that I had made the right decision. It felt like I had given myself space, space to think, space to write and to read, space to breathe. In a way, my year of being alone had prepared me for this situation, made it possible for me to retreat here and give myself the space for a kind of psychological convalescence, for easing the noise in my head, the volume of which I thought I had become accustomed to. It felt like an act of emancipation, an act of self-care. I would end up staying for two months.

'Self-care', of course, is a concept that has become ubiquitous today. It has become the defining contemporary approach to healing oneself, largely and thankfully replacing notions of self-optimization that had long dominated popular psychological discourses. Self-care today is anything but radical; it describes instead an elusive, in some respects problematic, smorgasbord of practices, ranging from spa treatments and social-media breaks to Ayurvedic and meditation retreats, as well as therapeutic interventions. It is so omnipresent today that one has to wonder if the reason that we celebrate self-care the way we do is because we can no longer do the very thing it aims to achieve: take care of ourselves in a comprehensive way.

My intuitive reaction to today's invocations of self-care is a negative one, not least because its commercialization rubs me up the wrong way. Fundamentally, I cannot help suspecting that it represents the ultimate victory of neoliberal late capitalism. We seem to have agreed to leave countless structural problems unresolved while taking on full responsibility for the resulting psychological consequences. Yet self-care is one of the most important aspects of my life: over the years, practising it has helped me time and again to accept things I did not want to accept and to find solutions to situations that seemed hopeless.

Surprisingly, the core concept of our contemporary concern for the self goes back, in large part, to the American poet, essayist and political activist Audre Lorde. Lorde, whose work I was rereading during those weeks, casually summed up her concept of self-care in the epilogue to her influential diary essay *A Burst of Light: Living with Cancer*. 'Caring for myself', she writes, 'is not self-indulgence, it is self-preservation, and that is an act of political warfare.'[2] She wrote down this much-quoted sentence three years after her second cancer diagnosis and five years before her death. She had survived breast cancer, but now a metastasis of the original tumour had formed in her liver. In her essay, the reader, silent, breath held, accompanies Lorde through this period of her life. You witness her despair and her affirmation of life; her grief, love and lust for life; learn how she uses all of the conventional, holistic and homeopathic remedies at her disposal, leaving no stone unturned in her fight against her illness; how she divides her energies, teaches, writes, meditates, reads and with what love she meets her partner Frances and their two children. One is impressed by the clarity and strength with which she confronts the racism that accosts her from all sides every day as a Black woman, the virulent misogyny and homophobia of the 1980s, the countless acts of resistance, moments of ostracism and discrimination that everyday life has in store for her.

In Lorde's beautiful and hard-earned life as a writer and activist – a life that society had not intended for her – self-care amounted to a form of 'self-preservation'. Self-preservation in a world hostile to her, her family and her community. By caring for herself, she expanded that hostile world to include a space that did not yet exist, a space where a life like hers could be lived and the power of the rampant fantasies of superiority that are masculinity, heterosexuality and white skin colour could be resisted, or at least put in check. This meant changing the world in small, enduring ways and making it a better place. It also meant living rather than just surviving. Self-care in this sense is an exceedingly radical idea.

AGAINST THE BACKDROP of the pandemic, Lorde's essay read differently. I felt connected to her in a new way and, faced with all the disease and death around us, I felt I better grasped her radicalism. I would get up early, read for a while, slice up a papaya or a pineapple for breakfast and write. I continued my daily walks, now along the island's sea cliffs overlooking a constantly stormy sea with sometimes gigantic waves. I started eating better and more healthily again, something I had completely neglected in the year leading up to my trip.

On the very first day of my stay, I had also bought a yoga mat. Like a lot of other people, yoga had helped me many times throughout my life. During personal crises, I had usually found my way back to a regular practice, but later, when I was feeling better again, I always stopped. When I rolled out my new mat on the floor of the apartment, I hadn't done yoga for over a year and a half. My body still remembered the backbends and stretches, all the asanas it had once performed, but it was no longer capable of doing them all. For some reason, though, I still managed to get my mat out every afternoon.

ALL PSYCHOLOGICAL WORK starts with the body. I knew that, had experienced it several times, but always forgot it again. When we talk about bodies, we almost always talk about their surfaces, what they look like, how to transform them and protect them from the effects of ageing. As British psychotherapist Susie Orbach points out, we understand our bodies today as something that we are meant to create, fabricate and optimize. We live in a cultural climate, says Orbach, in which perfecting our bodies is perceived as a personal duty, a kind of self-competence.[3] Much has happened in recent years to address this climate around the body and its virulent visual grammar. But even the critiques of problematic body images that we have internalized are still only really aimed at the body's surface, at liberating ourselves from the pressure to make our bodies more beautiful. What is forgotten in these discussions is the internal experience – what it is like to live in our bodies, to inhabit them, what emotional world they generate. However, as Olivia Laing argues in her book *Everybody*, which draws on the psychoanalytic theory of Wilhelm Reich, this is the experience that really matters, the experience that really counts.[4]

During my afternoon yoga practice, I kept thinking about the idea of the trauma body. Trauma researcher Bessel van der Kolk has argued in his seminal book *The Body Keeps the Score* that traumatic experiences leave their mark not only on our culture, our history, our families and of course our psyches, but also on the biochemical balance of our brains, on our bodies themselves. Trauma alters our ability to sense, process and deal with emotions, transforming neurological connections, hormonal processes, the rhythms of our hearts and the way our immune systems function. Trauma can deprive the body of its ability to sense itself, to be aware that it is alive. For van der Kolk, yoga is one of the ways in which we can get back in touch with our body, our organism. According to his observations, it helps us to do exactly what we often try and avoid, especially in difficult phases in our lives, and what the culturally conditioned view of the surfaces of our bodies prevents us from doing: to look inwards.[5]

I had a similar experience doing yoga on the island. Every afternoon, I followed the instructions and explanations of yoga teachers online for an hour and gave myself over to the flow of the asanas and to my breath. At first it was a huge challenge. Partly because I was out of shape, of course, but also because I shied away from looking inside, because I didn't seem able to cope with the sensations that the exercises evoked in me. But I stuck with it. The practice made me feel like I was getting to know my body all over again, a body that had not felt anything for so long, that had not been embraced or touched for so long, whose needs I had ignored for so long.

Each yoga session led to an improvement in my relationship with myself that was at first barely perceptible. The exercises forced me to accept my limitations and seemed to make me understand, again and again, that, in the end, even situations that are unpleasant and exhausting will eventually pass. And that one can still do something for one's inner balance, whatever challenges one is faced with. Gradually, my body began to open up on the mat, to take up space and release the tension, resistance and fear that were stored up in it, the uncertainties and traumas of the past year. Yoga does not promise a cure, a miraculous liberation of our psyches. But if you do it regularly, you will eventually find that you learn to look at your inner shadows, focus on where it hurts. After a few days and weeks, I experienced feelings of relaxation and gratitude on a more regular basis. Gratitude for this body that I was living in, for this life that I was leading, for the fact that all of this was possible here, despite the dramatic situation in the world.

THE LITERATURE OF the hermit and the great Robinsonades of modernity – from Thoreau's *Walden*, to Daniel Defoe's *Robinson Crusoe* itself, to Jean-Paul Sartre's quintessential novel of loneliness, *Nausea* – show that, in the final analysis, it is rarely the case that one is ever truly alone. Thoreau repeatedly conversed with hikers during his exile in the woods and went home once a week to be cooked for by his mother. Robinson even managed to find a companion on a remote Caribbean island onto whom he could project all of his colonial fantasies. And, once a week, Antoine Roquentin, Sartre's Existentialist poster boy, disappointed in love and gripped by a nausea about the world, slept wordlessly with the bar owner Françoise. For modern literary hermits, complete solitude, solitude in a comprehensive sense, is no longer possible. Fundamentally, it is not possible for any of us, no matter how much we long to retreat.

There is a certain comfort to be found in this. I learned some Spanish so that I could exchange a few words with the retail staff at the HiperDino supermarkets, as well as my landlady. The steady flow of emails didn't stop in the coastal town. I took part in my support group meetings via Zoom. The monthly French book club that had emerged from my French course also took place via Zoom during the pandemic. Of course, I was in regular contact with some of my friends. I was incredibly grateful that I had access to all of these means of communication: email, Zoom, social media. They alleviated my solitude and helped me cope with my everyday life on the island.

Of course, as the social scientist Sherry Turkle analyses in her books *Alone Together* and *Reclaiming Conversation*, these types of media are not without their dangers. According to Turkle, they can lead to us losing the ability to be relaxed when we are on our own and instead become accustomed to constant distraction and social stimulation. While they help us to have relationships, they also open up the possibility of keeping the people with whom we have these relationships at a distance, so that we demand less of each other and settle for less real compassion, less real attention, less real closeness. According to Turkle, contemporary means of communication often give us a sense of connection without confronting us with the real demands of friendship and intimacy.[6]

I believe that Turkle is both right and wrong. Her astute analyses have helped shape the discourses around our digital lifestyles because they describe aspects of our engagement with these technologies that we are all familiar with. But such analyses age as quickly as the technologies they analyse. The arguments eventually resemble those historical arguments about the dangers of reading novels when they were first popularized, of telephones and radios when they were introduced, or of television when it was invented. Each new communication technology has led to warnings that it was going to destroy everything that makes us human. In their day, all of these considerations were, to some extent, justified. But, with a little historical distance, it becomes clear that these fears do not describe our relationships to these technologies, but only capture the anxieties around the particular moment in which we integrate them into our everyday lives and first have to become competent at dealing with them.

The idea that digitally mediated relationships would eventually replace our real interpersonal relationships seemed almost absurd to me given our experiences in the pandemic. Almost all the people I spoke to on the phone or on Zoom made it clear that what they missed most were other people. Almost all of them, even if they were in relationships or were firmly ensconced in their everyday family lives, complained about a certain isolation, a certain loneliness, a self-evident longing to meet up with their friends again.

OVER THOSE TWO MONTHS, a certain kind of acceptance set in. I had the impression that I was able to face my loneliness and thus my neediness. I required this long period of self-imposed solitude to understand that I had no other choice. Not only during the exceptional situation of the pandemic, but in general.

It is probably true that the majority of us have no other choice. We probably all have to learn to accept this at some point, whether we resist it or not. It is something that philosophers like Odo Marquard certainly believe. According to Marquard, the crux of loneliness lies not in the pain it causes, but in our ability to deal with this pain, in our 'capacity for loneliness'.[7] For him, it is only in the 'strength to be alone', the 'capacity to endure isolation' and the 'art of living so as to experience loneliness positively' that it becomes truly possible to encounter oneself and other people.

The truth is that even painful emotions can gift us something. It is hard to see this at the time. When one is caught up in them and is doing everything one can to avoid them, one feels, of course, that one would be better off without them. But they often teach us things that we wouldn't otherwise have learnt. Loneliness, writes the psychologist Clark E. Moustakas, always contains something deeply positive, despite its horrors. Only the realization that we are alone in a fundamental sense, despite the people in our lives who love us, ensures that we become aware of ourselves.[8] Without this insight, we cannot take responsibility for ourselves and our lives, cannot build a good relationship with ourselves and really take care of ourselves. If we close ourselves off too much from our existential loneliness, Moustakas says, if we only repress and deny it, then we fence off an important path to inner growth.[9] The experience of loneliness, in other words, brings with it a form of self-awareness that we cannot otherwise attain. It is precisely the pain that accompanies it that allows us to uncover a new kind of compassion in ourselves, for ourselves and other people, that opens up new ways of living and allows us to deal with issues within ourselves in a way that would otherwise be impossible. Without this pain, we would not be able to seek closeness to other people, we would not be able to love.

Positive experiences of loneliness are as central to our humanity as the anguish this feeling causes. Christian mystics welcomed loneliness because, in their minds, it created a special closeness to their God. Michel de Montaigne also appreciated solitude. For him, it was the basis of a particularly intimate form of the interior monologue.[10] Many philosophers who followed in his footsteps thought that this form of solitary interior monologue was necessary to achieve any kind of self-knowledge. According to Hannah Arendt, without solitude there would be no *vita contemplativa*; indeed thinking itself would be inconceivable. As she wrote in her book *On the Life of the Mind*, it is only in the conscious withdrawal from our busy lives, in a withdrawal from the world, that a space emerges in which something like a 'quest for meaning' becomes possible and in which 'thinking self' can occur, a conversation with something 'invisible'.[11] And for Emmanuel Lévinas, it is only in the 'solitude of existing' that the possibility of breaking through the boundaries of the ego is revealed. Only through the experience of our existential solitude, according to the philosopher, can we truly come 'face-to-face' with another person and understand that this person, in their own humanity and otherness, cannot be appropriated by us, cannot even be fully understood. For Lévinas, without experiences of loneliness, people are not able to escape the limitations of their egos and enter into real relationships with other people.[12]

It was only during those two months on the island that I began to understand that this was more than just philosophical theory. My time there was marked by a degree of self-care that I had never before allowed myself. Unexpectedly, a certain sense of peace entered into my life. I enjoyed my little daily routines, the reading, writing and yoga, the long walks and the Spanish lessons in the evening, the island's barren nature, the blazing sun, the tempestuous Atlantic. I had the impression that I was learning something about myself, discovering a new side of myself.

And in a certain sense, I needed this phase of solitude to pierce through my own egotism, which I had not wanted or been able to see until then. My feelings of abandonment had been so defining that, whenever I thought about my friends, it always left me with a lingering sense of disappointment and reproach, with an underlying anger at being deserted by them at a time like this. No matter how much compassion I tried to muster for them, I could not accept the fact that I could not rely on them as much as I had always hoped. Nor could I accept that my wish to not feel alone was simply impossible to fulfil in these exceptional times.

I suddenly realized that I had been too focused on myself over the past months, that I had been too preoccupied with my own fears and problems, with my everyday life in the pandemic, to be genuinely receptive to the fears and problems that those people close to me were struggling with. And that they probably felt the same way. We were all trying, somehow, to cope with a situation that made it difficult for us to do just that and forced us to turn our internal spotlight back on ourselves. In doing so, we inevitably paid less attention to the lives of the people we loved. Not because we wanted to, not out of malice or because we were bad people, but simply because the world we lived in had changed so much that it suddenly became a necessity. It was only then that I grasped that I had disregarded perhaps the only basic rule of friendship: that friendships are based on freedom, not on social constraints or institutionalized obligations. Friends do not have to conform to one's own wishes, expectations and demands; one does not, in fact, have to demand anything from them. This remarkable freedom is the condition for our friendships to exist. I had disregarded what Jacques Derrida had described as the declaration of amicable love par excellence: 'I renounce you, I have decided to.'

BY THE END of my stay on the island, I felt better than I had in a long time. I could sense it in my body, that I was moving through the world with greater ease. Looking in the mirror on the morning of my departure, I noticed that my sun-tanned face looked a little narrower and its contours more prominent than when I had arrived. A few wrinkles had become visible around my eyes that I had not noticed before. I looked at them for a few minutes, contemplating their shape, tracing their course with my fingertips, trying to smooth them out. But gradually I noticed how my slight dismay increasingly gave way to a feeling of calm. The wrinkles did not bother me. They were signs of all those experiences, of all those startling changes, of all those psychological ups and downs of the past year. Traces of a reality that I had lived through, that had become an indelible part of my life. They suited my face. I found them beautiful.

Farewells

I returned to a spring that seemed unable to chase away the cold and dark of winter. The parks, streets and squares of Berlin still seemed to be doused in twilight, to be half asleep, but, in people's interactions, something seemed to be simmering away beneath the surface. Everyday encounters could trigger emotional responses that I didn't know how to deal with. People's sense of how to relate to one another seemed to have been collectively shaken. Everywhere you met people who knew better than anyone else how to defeat the pandemic once and for all. Everyone seemed to feel particularly disadvantaged by the political measures designed to tackle the still-vertiginous infection rates, believing that it was only their age group, only their family type or profession that had to bear the brunt of these changes. The spirited calls for 'solidarity' the year before had now largely disappeared from public discourse.

For the first time in history, vaccines against a dangerous virus had been developed in just one year. But instead of a sense of gratitude for this until recently unimaginable medical advance, there was a wide-spread frustration about the fact that a few countries were managing to vaccinate their populations faster. Everyone seemed to be so used to being among the most privileged people in the world that being relegated to second place seemed unbearable. But despite all this, a few glimmers of hope did manage to break through the cold and the grey spring clouds.

ON THE VERY FIRST DAY after I arrived, I inspected the plants on my terrace, freed them from their winter covers, fertilized and watered them, trimmed the bay and the yuzu trees and put them back outside together beside the variegated geraniums. To my relief, the large black bamboo had survived the harsh winter; some of its shoots had suffered frost damage, but it was covered in leaf buds, which would sprout in a few weeks' time. A few chervil and parsley leaves were already ready to be harvested; the tarragon, angelica and Swiss mint were sprouting; a few brave shiso seeds had sown themselves and were already germinating. The black cherry plum was covered with thick flower buds that would burst open in a few days and envelop the tree in a lavishly beautiful veil of soft, serene pink, ready to do battle with the Berlin sky.

I called Sylvia to find out how the garden in Wandlitz that I had helped her create a year and a half earlier was doing. Outside of the microclimate of the city, things seemed to be relatively quiet from a botanical point of view. But there, too, the change in the weather and the mood that the coming weeks would bring had already been heralded. The Lenten and Christmas roses were in full bloom; snowdrops had sprouted everywhere; the Indian yellow, cerulean blue and purple-striped crocuses that we had planted were blossoming.

Over the past year I had only been able to see the garden a few times and each of those occasions had made me very happy. Despite many problems, something had almost always been in bloom: from the winter-flowering honeysuckle, already displaying its first ivory-coloured flowers in January, to the last cosmoses, Japanese anemones and chrysanthemums of the year, which painted the greyish-brown Brandenburg November in bright rosy, lilac and crimson brushstrokes. The irises, tulips and Siberian buglosses had made marks that were almost impressionistic. The peonies, foxgloves and Heliopsis had unfolded their splendour; lush false goat's beard, phloxes, perennial sunflowers, perovskias, white gaura, tall grasses and large wild fennel plants had followed. The garden lived, grew and breathed. It was unfinished and beautiful.

SOME YEARS AGO, an acquaintance had tried to explain to me over and over again that one had to learn to live with unresolved problems. He said this so often and in so many different situations that it came to resemble a curious form of self-invocation that I couldn't comprehend. I believed that almost all problems could be solved if one tried hard enough, sought help, took the right steps, got involved. Maybe it was only now, in the pandemic, that I understood what he meant.

For Audre Lorde, this insight came when she was confronted with her cancer. 'One of the hardest things to accept', she wrote in *A Burst of Light*, 'is learning to live with uncertainty and neither deny nor hide behind it.' One must learn to listen to the 'messages of uncertainty' without being immobilized by them, she continues. The trick is not to settle into what has not yet happened, despite everything. Of course, you have to believe in a future in some way and work towards it, but it is only in the present that you can live your life to the fullest.[1]

Lorde's words and those of my acquaintance kept running through my head as spring really arrived. The cherry plum on my terrace faded and was replaced by the lilac, the mock orange and the pale-red umbels of the red-leaved elder. The pineapple sage, the lemon verbena, the signet marigold, the lovage and the lavender shot up; the geranium blossoms began to dance their radiant, delicate round that, if all went well, would last all summer. The city's trees were plunged into a dense bright green that made the idea that only a few weeks earlier everything had been bare seem almost amusing. The year entered its bucolic phase, in which every front garden, every flower bed, every park sank under luxuriant carpets of blossoms that enveloped you in a new cloud of fragrance wherever you strolled. It was now easy to get tested for the virus wherever you went, which made daily life much easier. Little by little, an increasing number of people received their first vaccinations, some already their second. I, too, was vaccinated for the first time and began to feel a little bit more secure while going about my daily life.

There was a sense of a new dawn, though it did not yet feel possible to say what this new era would bring. So many people had been sick. So many had been permanently impaired by the disease. So many had died. They were barely talked about in public, perhaps because their dying was too real to deal with. No one could really estimate how long the immunization from the vaccinations would last or how they would hold up against future variants of the virus. Most experts seemed to assume that a relatively relaxed summer lay ahead, but that afterwards the virus would keep causing new foci of infection, with smaller epidemics flaring up regionally. It was assumed that, as with influenza, vaccines would change annually. However, it was clear that at any time, a new, even more rapidly transmissible and deadly variant of the virus could shatter these predictions.

I went on long walks in the countryside around Berlin with Frederik, a friend I knew from New York who was going through a divorce. Sylvia came to Berlin and we went to our hairdresser's together, not far from the street where we had lived together many years ago. Kristof and Gunnar, a couple I'm friends with, picked me up from home and we walked along the Landwehrkanal and ate grilled chicken with *toum*, a Lebanese garlic sauce. Marie came over to help me assemble and hang a large mirrored cabinet for the bathroom that I had just purchased. I had bought it because I wanted to see myself more clearly in the morning, with my new wrinkles, my greying temples, my changing body. I made plans to visit my parents and siblings, started going to exhibitions again and looked forward to the reopening of the city's concert halls, operas, theatres and cinemas. I thought about what I was going to cook for the first dinner party I was going to host in over a year. Sometimes I managed to briefly smile back when men flirted with me in the street. I had started hugging people again.

IT WAS POSSIBLE to make out on the horizon the end of that period of liminality that the pandemic represented, the end of that limbo in which we found ourselves. You could sense, everywhere, a desire to forget the time that had past, to enjoy this new freedom and to act as if the pandemic had never happened at all. But every attempt to live out that desire only masked the beginning of a new era of uncertainty. There was no escaping the fact that whatever kind of 'return to normality' most of us wanted, it was unlikely to ever happen. We would have to learn to live with a problem that – despite the many successes in combating it – was, at its core, unresolved and likely to remain so.

In most wealthy countries, health systems had only just managed to meet the challenges of the virus. Elsewhere, the pandemic raged on inexorably, delivering wave after wave of death, spawning new variant after new variant. For a long time, Europe, America and China watched on, largely impassive, despite the fact that these variants would inevitably spread among their populations too. And this added to the fact that the destruction of natural habitats, the main cause of viral transmission from animals to humans, carried on apace. Sooner or later, a new epidemic might break out, with a virus that might be much less easy to control.

There were numerous other problems too that had preoccupied us before the pandemic and which had also not disappeared; indeed, they had intensified. The events of the past year and a half had fed the engine of neoliberal redistribution, responsible for so many of our social, economic and environmental hardships. While the majority of people became poorer, the richest in the world managed to profit from what had happened, increasing their fortunes to once-unimaginable new heights. A number of geopolitical flashpoints began to reignite. We ignored the fact that more and more people had to flee to other parts of the world, that everywhere forests were on fire again and rivers bursting their banks, that the rainforest continued to be decimated at record speed, that the hole in the ozone layer over Antarctica was suddenly widening again, that in Greenland the largest iceberg on record had detached from the mainland and that, according to most climate researchers, the dreaded tipping points had been reached, leading, irrevocably, to global warming with its extreme weather patterns, our vital ocean currents shifting, sea levels rising.

The liminality of the pandemic had protected us from the realization that we were already living in an era determined by what the anthropologist Árpád Szakolczai has aptly called 'permanent liminality'.[2] It became clear again that much of what we have taken for granted in our everyday lives would continue to disappear. That the much-vaunted 'end of normality' had already been set in motion many years ago. We were going through a transitional period, the outcome of which could not be foreseen and was beyond our comprehension. This feeling of permanent liminality is both a social and a personal problem. It upsets our inner ecology of affects and emotions, makes our lives feel paradoxical, creating a sense of unreality.[3] Despite the fact that my everyday life felt freer and lighter, this sense of paradox did not loosen its grip on me. I felt what Roland Barthes, in dialogue with psychoanalyst Donald Winnicott, described as the 'fear of what has happened', the fear of 'a catastrophe that has already occurred'.[4] I had the impression that my understanding was lagging behind what was happening, and that what I was afraid of had long since become a reality. I knew, and at the same time did not want to accept, that above all, the pandemic had given us a glimpse of the changes that awaited us in the future, that this glimpse had already cost us so much, demanded so much of us, and that it was far graver than a mere warning. The pandemic gave us an understanding of what it would look like, this end of the world whose narratives we have been familiar with for so long. In a sense, it was the catastrophe, it was the collapse that had already happened.

DURING THIS TIME, I was going through some old notes and came across a sheet of paper with a list I had made in therapy a few years back. The therapist had suggested I write out, in bullet points, how I imagined my own, very private future. This list included that I wanted to live in an old farmhouse near Berlin – not alone, but together with someone I loved, someone with whom I had endless conversations, someone whom I desired, with whom I shared my life. It was to be an open house; there would always be room for visitors and time for feasts. I would grow vegetables and fruits in the garden that were hard to buy elsewhere and that tasted so much better freshly harvested: mulberries, sour cherries, apricots and various kinds of peaches, cima di rapa, Castelfranco radicchio, borlotti beans. I would earn enough from my writing to build up a pension and live a quieter life. I would no longer constantly doubt the meaning of everything, my place in this life.

I stared at the sheet of paper entranced and read the points over and over again. Suddenly I understood that, in my hands, I was holding a very unambiguous list of my ambiguous losses. It detailed variations on desires and hopes that I had carried around for many years and that I had probably shared with many people. I held in my hands a testimony to what the writer Deborah Levy, in her book *Real Estate*, laconically refers to as her 'unreal estate', an illusory, fantasy property. In one of the most touching passages in this novelistic essay, Levy talks to a friend about her very own fantasy property, a house on a river, with a mooring and a boat, with pomegranate and mimosa trees, somewhere on the Mediterranean. All her life, she says, she has carried this house inside her. Her friend asks her if the weight of this fantasy is not too great, if it would not be better to let it go. Levy's answer was that she would collapse if she didn't have this house, collapse if there wasn't this future life to look forward to.[5] I understood what she meant.

I had long been sustained by this fantasy of a life with someone else in a big farmhouse with sweeping gardens. But a part of me knew, even then when I made that list, that I had already begun to grieve the ambiguous losses gathered together on that piece of paper. A few weeks later, I had broken off the therapy. One reason was the conversation about the list. The therapist had wanted me to feel that I could achieve this life if I just wanted it enough and worked hard enough for it. In a way, his goal was to re-establish in me that very thing that Lauren Berlant calls our 'cruel optimism'. I knew that one of the foundations of treatment for depression was instilling a sense of self-efficacy, a sense of being in control of one's own life, knew that the therapist was doing his job. And yet I felt that there was something illusory in this outlook. I had reached a point at which I had to put into perspective those expectations that were increasingly unlikely to ever become reality. Perhaps it was even time to say goodbye to them for good.

The therapist seemed unable to comprehend this. For him, his view of the world felt right; it had been confirmed to him again and again. He was, in fact, convinced that we can all control our lives and realize our dreams, at least for the most part. I knew people like him. I had friends and acquaintances like him. They assumed that what they wished for would, to all intents and purposes, come true. They could not grasp that they could only maintain this belief because they were privileged. That one only had this belief confirmed over and over again if one came from a certain social class and certain parts of the country, had a certain skin colour and a certain sexual orientation, if one had certain biographical and psychological prerequisites. I did not belong to these people; nor, anymore, did I want to.

The question that ran through my head as I read the points on the list over and over again was who I might be without them. What might my life look like if I were not trying to realize these fantasies? Pauline Boss, who spent so many years exploring how we deal with ambiguous loss, found again and again that people are surprisingly resilient. One of the central messages of her work is that we can succeed in living with the ambivalence that defines our existence.

Sometimes, says Boss, solutions to our problems simply cannot be found because these solutions do not exist. Sometimes ambiguity cannot be dealt with or treated. Sometimes pressing questions remain unanswered because they have no answer. Our task then is to accept this ambiguity and, in this acceptance, to look for new possibilities for ourselves. Even though ambiguous losses can be traumatic, we are still able to shape our lives, live them fully and find contentment. For Boss, this had nothing to do with passivity, with stoicism or adaptation, but with establishing a certain inner freedom.[6] We go through life with the assumption that we have to 'get over' everything. Often that's exactly what doesn't work; often, in order to find our way, it is precisely this assumption that we have to get over.

MY FAVOURITE GARDEN, by the way, the garden that touches me most, is not by Piet Oudolf, whom I admire so much. Nor does it radiate the classical beauty of the gardens of Jean-Baptiste de la Quintinie, Karl Foerster or Vita Sackville-West. It is in Dungeness, in Kent, two hours southeast of London, not far from a nuclear power station that dominates that flat coastal landscape. It is only a few hundred yards from a stony beach on the English Channel and belongs to a small house called Prospect Cottage, made of black-stained wood with neon-yellow window frames. The garden was created by the gay painter and filmmaker Derek Jarman. I had visited it with Andrew, a friend from London, the year before the pandemic.

Jarman came across Prospect Cottage by chance in 1986 while doing research for a film. He already had contracted HIV, the disease that would kill him almost eight years later.[7] The conditions for gardening in Dungeness were highly challenging. The landscape was barren, the stony ground was too dry and too nutrient-poor for most garden plants; briny easterly winds and strong sunlight burnt their leaves. With the help of a friend, Jarman carted in manure, improved the soil, built raised beds and beehives behind the house, experimented with different varieties of plants and found out what kind of protection they needed from the adverse weather conditions there. What began with a frail dog rose and the indestructible accidental seedling of a red-leaved sea kale developed over the years into a remarkably beautiful garden in which blossomed gorse, marigolds, tea roses, Lenten roses, hollyhocks, poppies, lavender, hyssop, acanthus, fennel, caraway and a small fig tree. Among the plants were sculptures Jarman had created from driftwood, metal objects and stones that he had found during his walks on the beach.

Jarman's passion for this project had much to do with his illness and approaching death. But Prospect Cottage was not only a symbol of his life as a gay man under the most adverse social conditions; it was a symbol of so much more. In *Modern Nature*, his diary of the last few years of his life, he describes how he had chained himself to the inhospitable coastal landscape and how his garden saved him time and again from the whole 'demon Disney World' in which he was living. The AIDS crisis, forest dieback, the hole in the ozone layer, the greenhouse effect, the Chernobyl disaster, the nuclear threat at the height of the Cold War – all of these things created in him a sense of impending apocalypse. He took a few seeds, some cuttings and some driftwood and began to transform this feeling of the end of the world into art, thus alleviating its horror.[8]

I knew of no better example of how to live with those problems that cannot be solved, with questions for which there are no answers. Jarman had created meaning in a world that had lost its meaning, confidence in an age that knew little of it. He had, to paraphrase Audre Lorde, listened to the messages of uncertainty that defined his life without being immobilized or intimidated by them. He took full advantage of the here and now. In the shadow of a nuclear power station and in the shadow of his approaching death, he managed to brace himself against the ambiguity of the future and to bid farewell to many of the ambiguous losses of his life. I wondered if, under different circumstances and on a different scale, I might not be able to attempt something similar.

I WAS STILL HOLDING my list of future fantasies for a life with a partner in a pastoral property. It was written on a page I had torn out of one of the unassuming legal pads I bring back from my visits to the States because I like their colour so much. Neapolitan yellow with light-blue lines, a thin, vertical red line to denote the margin. The even arcs of my handwriting on the surface, in indigo blue.

In between all the stories we tell ourselves in order to live, and in between all of our attempts to discard those stories when we realize that they are distorting our view of things and that they are becoming prisons of our own making, there are moments of stillness. I had the impression that I was experiencing just such a moment. They are moments of great openness, when everything seems possible and impossible at the same time. Moments of confusion, of disappointment and optimism, of not knowing and of not having to know. They are moments in which, sometimes, without realizing it, you take a step forward and move in a new direction. It is in precisely these moments that life rewrites itself.

I had to think of all those people who had accompanied me through my life and wondered how they would fit into my future in this big house. Of all those people I loved in my own way and who loved me in their own way, likeable, kind, quirky, exhausting, clever, demanding, fascinating and damaged people who went through life despite briny easterly winds and burning sunshine. People I could sometimes rely on and sometimes not, who left me alone and yet accompanied me, helped me through the days and made my life, this life alone, possible in the first place. People with whom I wanted to share my future and with whom I would share it.

PERHAPS THIS IS WHAT the philosopher Simone Weil meant when she described the existence of friendships as a 'miracle', as 'a miracle, like the beautiful'.⁹ Friendships and the balancing act they perform between closeness and distance were, for her, a prime example of how we might live with ambiguity. The fact that friendships exist despite their inherent uncertainty was, to her, like a gift, a grace.¹⁰ This may sound full of pathos, but for Weil it was an insight that she had wrung out from her hard, often-lonely life between the wars, a life rich in historic catastrophes. A life in which it looked more than once as if the world was about to stop turning, as if there would be no future.

I thought long and hard about what to do with the list in my hand. I was already on my way to the kitchen to throw it into the bin with the rest of the waste paper. But then I turned back. Without being able to say why, I smoothed it out and put it back with my notes.

NOTES

Unless otherwise specified, translations from the German are the translator's own.

Living Alone

1 Anthony Feinstein and Hannah Storm, 'The Emotional Toll on Journalists Covering the Refugee Crisis', report by the Reuters Institute for the Study of Journalism, July 2017; see also Nicole Krauss, 'We're Living in a World of Walls: Here Is a Window to Escape', in *New York Times* (23 October 2020).

2 On the psychologically beneficial side effects of gardening, see Sue Stuart-Smith, *The Well Gardened Mind: Rediscovering Nature in the Modern World* (London, 2020).

3 See Jean-François Lyotard, *The Postmodern Condition: A Report on Knowledge*, trans. Geoff Bennington and Brian Massumi (Manchester, 1984).

4 Eva Illouz, *Why Love Hurts: A Sociological Explanation* (Cambridge, 2013), and also *The End of Love: A Sociology of Negative Relationships* (New York, 2019).

5 Julia Samuel, *This Too Shall Pass: Stories of Change, Crisis and Hopeful Beginnings* (London, 2020), p. 113.

6 Sasha Roseneil, 'Neue Freundschaftspraktiken. Fürsorge und Sorge um sich im Zeitalter der Individualisierung', in *Mittelweg 36: Zeitschrift des Hamburger Instituts für Sozialforschung* (*Journal of the Hamburg Institute of Social*

Research), XVII/3 (June/July 2008), pp. 55–70 and specifically pp. 58–60.

7 The exact figures for Germany can be found in 'Bevölkerung und Erwerbstätigkeit: Haushalte und Familien. Ergebnisse des Mikrozensus', Federal Statistical Office (Destatis), 11 July 2019 – 17.3 million people in Germany live in a single-person household. This number has increased by almost 50 per cent since the early 1990s and accounts for 42 per cent of total households. Two-person households account for only 34 per cent of households, and there are even fewer three- and four-person households. A similar situation prevails in almost all Western European countries as well as North America.

8 For the scientific rationale for why close ties are the most effective means of countering emotional distress, see Amir Levine and Rachel Heller, *Attached* (London, 2019), and Giovanni Frazzetto, *Together, Closer: The Art and Science of Intimacy in Friendship, Love and Family* (New York, 2017).

9 Marilyn Friedman, 'Freundschaft und moralisches Wachstum', *Deutsche Zeitschrift für Philosophie*, XLV/2 (January 1997), pp. 235–48, here p. 235.

10 Roseneil, 'Neue Freundschaftspraktiken', pp. 62 and 67.

11 See Liz Spencer and Ray Pahl, *Rethinking Friendship: Hidden Solidarities Today* (Princeton, NJ, and Oxford, 2006).

12 See Janosch Schobin, Vincenz Leuschner, Sabine Flick, Erika Alleweldt, Eric Anton Heuser and Agnes Brandt, *Freundschaft heute: Eine Einführung in die Freundschaftssoziologie* (Bielefeld, 2016), pp. 11–19.

13 For a detailed breakdown of the spectrum of friendship, see Spencer and Pahl, *Rethinking Friendship*, pp. 59–107.

14 Maggie Nelson, *The Red Parts: Autobiography of a Trial* (London, 2015), p. 155.

15 Robert Harrison, *Gardens: An Essay on the Human Condition* (Chicago, IL, 2008).

The Kindness of Strangers

1 Roland Barthes, *Roland Barthes by Roland Barthes*, trans. Richard Howard (New York, 2010).

2 Maggie Nelson, *Bluets* (London, 2017).

3 Marguerite Duras, *Writing*, trans. Mark Polizzotti (Minneapolis, MN, 2011), pp. 26–7.

4 Lauren Berlant, *Cruel Optimism* (Durham and London, 2011), pp. 1–21.

5 Ibid., p. 187.

6 Ibid., p. 14.

7 Roland Barthes, *A Lover's Discourse: Fragments*, trans. Richard Howard (London, 2018), pp. 212–13.

8 Virginia Woolf, *Street Haunting: A London Adventure* (San Francisco, CA, 1930), pp. 2–3.

9 On the philosophy and history of walking, see Rebecca Solnit, *Wanderlust: A History of Walking* (London, 2014).

10 On the concept of idiosyncrasy, see Silvia Bovenschen, *Über-Empfindlichkeit. Spielformen der Idiosynkrasie* (Frankfurt am Main, 2000), especially the chapter 'Ach wie schön: Freundschaft und idiosynkratische Befremdungen', pp. 119–49.

11 A description of the everyday meaning of this 'web of friends' that feels very authentic can be found in Ann Friedman and Aminatou Sow, *Big Friendship: How We Keep Each Other Close* (New York, 2020), especially pp. 99–117.

12 Mark S. Granovetter, 'The Strength of Weak Ties', *American Journal of Sociology*, LXXVIII/6 (May 1973), pp. 1360–80.

13 For example, Nicholas A. Christakis and James H. Fowler, *Connected: The Surprising Power of Social Networks and How They Shape Our Lives* (New York and London, 2009), or Lydia Denworth, *Friendship: The Evolution, Biology, and Extraordinary Power of Life's Fundamental Bond* (New York, 2020), especially pp. 138–63.

14 Adam Philips and Barbara Taylor, *On Kindness* (London, 2009).

15 A thoroughly stimulating philosophy-of-life approach to kindness can be found in The School of Life, *On Being Nice* (London, 2017).

Conversations with Friends

1 Silvia Bovenschen, 'Vom Tanz der Gedanken und Gefühle', in Juliane Beckmann and Silvia Bovenschen, eds, *Von der Freundschaft. Ein Lesebuch* (Frankfurt am Main, 2009), pp. 7–18, here p. 12.

2 Hans-Georg Gadamer, 'Freundschaft und Selbsterkenntnis: Zur Rolle der Freundschaft in der griechischen Ethik' (1985), in *Gesammelte Werke*, Vol. VII (Tübingen, 1999), pp. 396–406, here p. 405.

3 Hans-Georg Gadamer, 'Freundschaft und Solidarität', in *Hermeneutische Entwürfe: Vorträge und Aufsätze* (Tübingen, 2000), pp. 56–65, here p. 56.

4 Gilles Deleuze and Felix Guattari, *What Is Philosophy?*, trans. Graham Burchell and Hugh Tomlinson (New York, 1996).

5 Alexander Nehamas, *On Friendship* (New York, 2016).

6 Aristotle, *Nicomachean Ethics*, Book VIII, Paragraph 2.

7   Aristotle, *Nicomachean Ethics*, Book IX, Paragraph 4.

8   Andree Michaelis-König and Erik Schilling, 'Poetik und Praxis der Freundschaft. Zur Einführung', in *Poetik und Praxis der Freundschaft (1800–1933)* (Heidelberg, 2019), pp. 9–23, here p. 13.

9   Andreas Schinkel, 'Das Selbst im Spiegel des Anderen. Zur Geschichte und Struktur der Freundschaft', in Dirk Villány, Matthias D. Witte and Uwe Sander, eds, *Globale Jugend und Jugendkulturen. Aufwachsen im Zeitalter der Globalisierung* (Weinheim and Munich, 2007), pp. 315–29, here p. 318.

10 Michel de Montaigne, *Montaigne's Essays in Three Books. With Notes and Quotations. And an Account of the Author's Life. With a Short Character of the Author and Translator, by the Late Marquiss of Hallifax*, trans. Charles Cotton (London, 1743), Chapter XXVII.

11 Ibid.

12 See Michael Monsour, 'The Hackneyed Notions of Adult "Same Sex" and "Opposite-Sex" Friendships', in Mahzad Hojjat and Anne Moyer, *The Psychology of Friendship* (Oxford, 2016), pp. 59–74.

13 Jacques Derrida, *The Politics of Friendship*, trans. George Collins (London, 2006), pp. 92 and 276.

14 See Marilyn Yalom with Theresa Donovan Broen, *The Social Sex: A History of Female Friendship* (New York, 2015).

15 Katrin Berndt, *Narrating Friendship and the British Novel, 1760–1830* (Oxford and New York, 2016).

16 See the influential study by Lillian Faderman, *Surpassing the Love of Men: Romantic Friendship and Love Between Women from the Renaissance to the Present* (New York, 1981).

17 Mitja D. Back, Stefan C. Schmukle and Boris Egloff, 'Becoming Friends by Chance', *Psychological Science*, XIX/5 (May 2008), pp. 439–40.

18 Maarten Selfhout et al., 'In the Eye of the Beholder: Perceived, Actual, and Peer-Rated Similarity in Personality, Communication, and Friendship Intensity During the Acquaintanceship Process', *Journal of Personality and Social Psychology*, XCVI/6 (June 2009), pp. 1152–65.

19 For example, Nicholas A. Christakis, *Blueprint: The Evolutionary Origin of Good Society* (New York, 2019), pp. 254f.

20 Klaus-Dieter Eichler, 'Zu einer Philosophie der Freundschaft' in *Philosophie der Freundschaft* (Leipzig, 1999), pp. 215–41, here p. 225.

21 See also Jon Nixon, *Hannah Arendt and the Politics of Friendship* (London and New York, 2015), pp. 159–75.

22 Matthias Bormuth, 'Im Spiegel Lessings oder Eine Republik der Freunde', in *Hannah Arendt: Freundschaft in finsteren Zeiten – Gedanken zu Lessing. Die Lessing-Rede mit Erinnerungen von Richard Bernstein, Mary McCarthy, Alfred Kazi und Jerome Kohn*, ed. and intro. Matthias Bormuth (Berlin, 2018).

23 Hannah Arendt, 'On Humanity in Dark Times: Thoughts about Lessing', in *Men in Dark Times* (London, 1970), p. 27.

24 Richard Riess, 'Freundschaft: Ferment des Lebens', in *Freundschaft*, ed. Richard Riess (Darmstadt, 2014).

25 Derrida, *The Politics of Friendship*, p. 174.

Never So Lonely

1 On this distinction, see Lars Svendsen, *A Philosophy of Loneliness* (London, 2017), p. 15.

2 Ibid., p. 22.

3 For example, David Riesman, *The Lonely Crowd: A Study of the Changing American Character* (Chicago, IL, 1950); Robert Putnam, *Bowling Alone: The Collapse and Survival of American Community* (New York, 2000); Vivek Murthy, *Together: The Healing Power of Human Connection in a Sometimes Lonely World* (New York, 2020); or most recently Diana Kinnert and Marc Bielefeld, *Die neue Einsamkeit. Und wie wir sie als Gesellschaft überwinden können* (Hamburg, 2021).

4 A good list of recent studies can be found here: Kerry Banks, 'Loneliness: The Silent Killer', University Affairs, 27 February 2019.

5 See George E. Vaillant, *The Men of the Harvard Grant Study* (London, 2012), pp. 27–53.

6 Olivia Laing, *The Lonely City: Adventures in the Art of Being Alone* (Edinburgh and London, 2016), p. 25.

7 Robert Weiss, *Loneliness: The Experience of Emotional and Social Isolation* (Boston, MA, 1975), p. 12.

8 Frieda Fromm-Reichmann, 'Loneliness', *Contemporary Psychoanalysis* (1959), XXVI/2 (1990), pp. 305–29, see especially pp. 313f.

9 Ibid.

10 Robert Weiss, *Loneliness: The Experience of Emotional and Social Isolation* (Boston, 1975), p. 11.

11 Giovanni Frazzetto, *Together, Closer: The Art and Science of Intimacy in Friendship, Love, and Family* (New York, 2017). Excerpt published in Gigi Falk, 'The True Cost of Loneliness', Thrive Global, https://thriveglobal.com, 11 July 2017.

12 Melanie Klein, 'On the Sense of Loneliness (1963)', in *Envy and Gratitude and Other Works, 1946–1963 (The Writings of Melanie Klein)* (London, 1984), pp. 300–313.

Ambiguous Losses

1 Victor Turner, *The Ritual Process: Structure and Anti-Structure* (Piscataway, NJ, 1996).

2 Pauline Boss, 'Ambiguous Loss Theory: Challenges for Scholars and Practitioners', *Family Relations*, LVI/2 (April 2007), pp. 105–12; see also Pauline Boss, *Loss, Trauma, and Resilience: Therapeutic Work with Ambiguous Loss* (New York, 2006).

3 See Hannah Black, 'The Loves of Others', *The New Inquiry*, https://thenewinquiry.com, 22 June 2018.

4 Ibid.

5 Lauren Berlant, *Desire/Love* (Brooklyn, NY, 2012), p. 69.

6 Zygmunt Bauman, *Liquid Love. On the Frailty of Human Bonds* (Cambridge, 2003), pp. viiif.

7 On these terms, see Patrick Carnes, *Sexual Anorexia: Overcoming Sexual Self-Hatred* (Center City, PA, 1997), and Douglas Weiss, *Intimacy Anorexia: Healing the Hidden Addiction in Your Marriage* (Colorado Springs, CO, 2010).

8 Janosch Schobin, 'Sechs Farben und drei Rotationsachsen: Versuch über Verpflichtungen in Freundschaften', *Mittelweg 36: Zeitschrift des Hamburger Instituts für Sozialforschung* (Journal of the Hamburg Institute of Social Research), XVII/2 (June/July 2008), pp. 17–41, citations pp. 36 and 38.

9 On the history and philosophy of knitting, see also Loretta Napoleoni, *The Power of Knitting: Stitching Together Our Lives in a Fractured World* (New York, 2020); Richard Rutt, *A History of Hand Knitting* (New York, 1989); and Ann Patchett, 'How Knitting Saved My Life: Twice', in *Knitting Yarns: Writers on Knitting*, ed. Ann Hood (New York and London, 2014), pp. 204–11.

10 Turner, *The Ritual Process*.

11 Ibid, p. 204. See also the epilogue by Eugene Rochberg-Halton.

12 Pauline Boss and Donna Carnes, 'The Myth of Closure', *Family Process*, LI/4 (December 2012), pp. 456–70.

Days in Famara

1 Roland Barthes, *How to Live Together: Novelistic Simulations of Some Everyday Spaces*, trans. Kate Briggs (New York, 2012).

2 Roland Barthes, *Mourning Diary: October 26, 1977–September 15, 1979*, trans. Richard Howard (New York, 2012), p. 178.

3 Walt Odets, *Out of the Shadows: Reimagining Gay Men's Lives* (New York, 2019), pp. 221–5.

4 Eve Kosofsky Sedgwick, 'Shame, Theatricality, and Queer Performativity: Henry James's *The Art of the Novel*', in David M. Halperin and Valerie Traub, *Gay Shame* (Chicago, IL, and London, 2009), pp. 49–62.

5 Alan Downs, *The Velvet Rage: Overcoming the Pain of Growing Up Gay in a Straight Man's World* (Cambridge, 2005), see, among others, the chapter 'Compensating for Shame', pp. 71–106.

6 Didier Eribon, *Insult and the Making of the Gay Self*, trans. Michael Lucey (Durham, NC, 2004).

7 On the history of the treatment of queerness, see, among others Benno Altman and Jonathan Symons, *Queer Wars* (Cambridge, 2016); Lillian Faderman, *The Gay Revolution: The Story of the Struggle* (New York, 2015); and Benno Gammerl, *Anders fühlen: Schwules und lesbisches Leben in der Bundesrepublik – Eine Emotionsgeschichte* (Munich, 2021).

8 Pierre Bourdieu, 'Le Mort saisit le vif: Les Relations entre l'histoire réifiée et l'histoire incorporée', *Actes de la recherche en sciences sociales*, 32 (1980).

9 Roxane Gay, *Hunger: A Memoir of (My) Body* (New York, 2017), p. 37.

10 For a description of this dystopia, see, for example, the wonderful essay 'Loneliness in the Age of Grindr' by the Indigenous Canadian author Billy-Ray Belcourt, in *A History of My Brief Body* (Columbus, OH, 2020), pp. 59–67.

11 See Michel Foucault, 'Friendship as a Way of Life', in *Ethics*, ed. Paul Rabinow, trans. Robert Hurley et al. (New York, 1994), pp. 135–56; see also the biographical study of the complicated friendships in Foucault's life: Tom Roach, *Friendship as a Way of Life: Foucault, AIDS and the Politics of Shared Estrangement* (New York, 2012).

12 Eribon, *Insult and the Making of the Gay Self*, pp. 25f.

Bodywork

1 Jacques Derrida, *The Politics of Friendship*, trans. George Collins (London, 2006).

2 Audre Lorde, *A Burst of Light and Other Essays* (Mineola, NY, 2017), p. 140.

3 Susie Orbach, *Bodies* (London, 2010).

4 Olivia Laing, *Everybody: A Book About Freedom* (London, 2021), see especially the introduction.

5 Bessel van der Kolk, *The Body Keeps the Score: Mind, Brain and Body in the Transformation of Trauma* (New York, 2015). See, for instance, his tremendously illuminating explanations of yoga practice and its psychological effects on pp. 263–74.

6 Sherry Turkle, *Alone Together: Why We Expect More from Technology and Less from Each Other* (New York, 2011); and Sherry Turkle, *Reclaiming Conversation: The Power of Talk in a Digital Age* (New York, 2015).

7 Odo Marquard, 'Plädoyer für die Einsamkeitsfähigkeit', in
   Skepsis und Zustimmung: Philosophische Studien (Stuttgart,
   1995), pp. 110–22.

8 See Clark A. Moustakas, *Loneliness* (Englewood Cliffs, NJ,
   1961); and Ben Lazare Mijuskovic, *Loneliness in Philosophy,
   Psychology and Literature* (New York, London and Amsterdam,
   1979), especially the chapter 'Loneliness and a Theory of
   Consciousness'.

9 Moustakas, *Loneliness*.

10 Michel de Montaigne, *Montaigne's Essays in Three Books. With
   Notes and Quotations. And an Account of the Author's Life. With
   A Short Character of the Author and Translator, by The Late
   Marquiss of Hallifax*, trans. Charles Cotton (London, 1743),
   chap. XXXVIII.

11 Hannah Arendt, *The Life of the Mind*, ed. Mary McCarthy
   (San Diego, New York and London, 1971), pp. 75–85.

12 Emmanuel Lévinas, *Time and the Other*, trans. Richard A.
   Cohen (Pittsburgh, PA, 2003).

Farewells

1 Audre Lorde, *The Selected Works of Audre Lorde*, ed. and
   intro. Roxane Gay (New York, 2020), p. 163.

2 Árpád Szakolczai, *Reflexive Historical Sociology* (London,
   2000), pp. 2017–217; and Árpád Szakolczai, 'Permanent
   (Trickster) Liminality: The Reasons of the Heart and
   of the Mind', *Theory and Psychology*, XXVII/2 (April 2017),
   pp. 231–48.

3 On these topics, see also Bjørn Thomassen, *Liminality and
   the Modern: Living Through the In-Between* (Farnham and
   Burlington, VT, 2014).

4 Roland Barthes, *Mourning Diary: October 26, 1977–September 15, 1979*, trans. Richard Howard (New York, 2012).

5 Deborah Levy, *Real Estate* (London, 2021), p. 83.

6 Pauline Boss, *Loss, Trauma, and Resilience: Therapeutic Work with Ambiguous Loss* (New York, 2006). See especially the section 'Therapeutic Goals for Treating Ambiguous Loss', pp. 71–210.

7 On the genesis of the garden, see Derek Jarman, *Derek Jarman's Garden*, photog. Howard Sooley (London, 1996).

8 Derek Jarman, *Modern Nature: The Journals of Derek Jarman, 1989–1990*, intro. Olivia Laing (London, 2018).

9 Simone Weil, *Gravity and Grace*, trans. Emma Crawford and Mario von der Rurh (London and New York, 2002).

10 Simone Weil, *Amitié. L'Art de bien aimer* (Paris, 2016). See the shrewd preface by Valérie Gérard, pp. 7–24.

BIBLIOGRAPHY

Altman, Benno, and Jonathan Symons, *Queer Wars* (Cambridge, 2016)

Arendt, Hannah, *The Life of the Mind*, ed. Mary McCarthy (San Diego, CA, New York and London, 1971)

—, 'On Humanity in Dark Times: Thoughts about Lessing', in *Men in Dark Times* (London, 1970)

—, and Matthias Bormuth, eds, *Freundschaft in finsteren Zeiten: Gedanken zu Lessing – Die Lessing-Rede mit Erinnerungen von Richard Bernstein, Mary McCarthy, Alfred Kazi und Jerome Kohn* (Berlin, 2018)

Aristotle, *The Nicomachean Ethics*, trans. J.A.K. Thomson, revd and n. Hugh Tredennick (London, 2004)

Back, Mitja D., Stefan C. Schmukle and Boris Egloff, 'Becoming Friends by Chance', *Psychological Science*, V/19 (May 2008), pp. 439–40

Badiou, Alain, with Nicolas Truong, *In Praise of Love*, trans. Peter Bush (London, 2012)

Barthes, Roland, *How to Live Together: Novelistic Simulations of Some Everyday Spaces*, trans. Kate Briggs (New York, 2012)

—, *Roland Barthes by Roland Barthes*, trans. Richard Howard (New York, 2010)

—, *Mourning Diary: October 26, 1977–September 15, 1979*, trans. Richard Howard (New York, 2012)

—, *A Lover's Discourse: Fragments*, trans. Richard Howard (London, 2018)

Bauman, Zygmunt, *Liquid Love: On the Frailty of Human Bonds* (Cambridge, 2003)

Belcour, Billy-Ray, *A History of My Brief Body* (Columbus, OH, 2020)

Berlant, Lauren, *Cruel Optimism* (Durham and London, 2011)

—, *Desire/Love* (Brooklyn, NY, 2012)

Berndt, Katrin, *Narrating Friendship and the British Novel, 1760–1830* (Oxford and New York, 2016)

Bernstein Sycamore, Mattilda, ed., *Why Are Faggots So Afraid of Faggots? Flaming Challenges to Masculinity, Objectification, and the Desire to Conform* (Oakland, CA, Edinburgh and Baltimore, MD, 2012)

Black, Hannah, 'The Loves of Others', *New Inquiry*, https://thenewinquiry.com, 22 June 2018

Bormuth, Matthias, 'Im Spiegel Lessings oder Eine Republik der Freunde', in *Hannah Arendt: Freundschaft in finsteren Zeiten – Gedanken zu Lessing. Die Lessing-Rede mit Erinnerungen von Richard Bernstein, Mary McCarthy, Alfred Kazi und Jerome Kohn*, ed. and intro. Matthias Bormuth (Berlin, 2018)

Boss, Pauline, *Loss, Trauma, and Resilience: Therapeutic Work with Ambiguous Loss* (New York, 2006)

—, and Donna Carnes, 'The Myth of Closure', *Family Process*, IV/51 (December 2012), pp. 456–70

Bourdieu, Pierre, 'Le Mort saisit le vif: Les Relations entre l'histoire réifiée et l'histoire incorporée', *Actes de la recherche en sciences sociales*, 32 (1980)

Bovenschen, Silvia, *Über-Empfindlichkeit: Spielformen der Idiosynkrasie* (Frankfurt am Main, 2000)

—, 'Vom Tanz der Gedanken und Gefühle', in Juliane Beckmann and Silvia Bovenschen, eds, *Von der Freundschaft: Ein Lesebuch* (Frankfurt am Main, 2009), pp. 7–18

Braun, Christina von, *Blutsbande: Verwandtschaft als Kulturgeschichte* (Berlin, 2018)

Brookner, Anita, *Hotel du Lac* (London, 1994)

Carnes, Patrick, *Sexual Anorexia: Overcoming Sexual Self-Hatred* (Center City, PA, 1997)

Christakis, Nicholas A., *Blueprint: The Evolutionary Origin of Good Society* (New York, 2019)

—, and James H. Fowler, *Connected: The Surprising Power of Social Networks and How They Shape Our Lives* (New York and London, 2009)

Deleuze, Gilles, and Felix Guattari, *What Is Philosophy?*, trans. Graham Burchell and Hugh Tomlinson (New York, 1996)

Denworth, Lydia, *Friendship: The Evolution, Biology, and Extraordinary Power of Life's Fundamental Bond* (New York, 2020)

Jacques Derrida, *The Politics of Friendship*, trans. George Collins (London, 2006)

Didion, Joan, *The Year of Magical Thinking* (New York, 2005)

—, *Slouching towards Bethlehem: Essays* (New York, 2008)

—, *The White Album: Essays* (New York, 2009)

Downs, Alan, *The Velvet Rage: Overcoming the Pain of Growing Up Gay in a Straight Man's World* (Cambridge, 2005)

Duras, Marguerite, *Writing*, trans. Mark Polizzotti (Minneapolis, MN, 2011)

Eichler, Klaus-Dieter, 'Zu einer Philosophie der Freundschaft', in
 Klaus-Dieter Eichler, ed., *Philosophie der Freundschaft* (Leipzig,
 1999), pp. 215–41
Eribon, Didier, *Insult and the Making of the Gay Self*, trans. Michael
 Lucey (Durham, NC, 2004)
Ernaux, Annie, *The Years*, trans. Alison L. Strayer (London, 2021)
Faderman, Lillian, *Surpassing the Love of Men: Romantic Friendship
 and Love Between Women from the Renaissance to the Present*
 (New York, 1981)
—, *The Gay Revolution: The Story of the Struggle* (New York, 2015)
Feinstein, Anthony, and Hannah Storm, *The Emotional Toll on
 Journalists Covering the Refugee Crisis*, Reuters Institute for the
 Study of Journalism (July 2017)
Fink, Bruce, *Lacan on Love: An Exploration of Lacan's Seminar VIII,
 Transference* (Cambridge, 2016)
Foucault, Michel, 'Friendship as a Way of Life', in *Ethics*, ed. Paul
 Rabinow, trans. Robert Hurley et al. (New York, 1994),
 pp. 135–56
Frazzetto, Giovanni, *Together, Closer: The Art and Science of Intimacy
 in Friendship, Love, and Family* (New York, 2017)
Friedman, Marilyn, 'Freundschaft und moralisches Wachstum',
 Deutsche Zeitschrift für Philosophie, XLV/2 (January 1997),
 pp. 235–48
Fromm-Reichmann, Frieda, 'Loneliness' (1959), *Contemporary
 Psychoanalysis*, XXVI/2 (1990), pp. 305–29
Gadamer, Hans-Georg, 'Freundschaft und Selbsterkenntnis: Zur
 Rolle der Freundschaft in der griechischen Ethik (1985)', in
 Gesammelte Werke, vol. VII (Tübingen, 1999), pp. 396–406
—, 'Freundschaft und Solidarität', in *Herme-neutische Entwürfe:
 Vorträge und Aufsätze* (Tübingen, 2000), pp. 56–65

Gammerl, Benno, *Anders fühlen: Schwules und lesbisches Leben in der Bundesrepublik – Eine Emotionsgeschichte* (Munich, 2021)

Gay, Roxane, *Hunger: A Memoir of (My) Body* (New York, 2017)

Granovetter, Mark S., 'The Strength of Weak Ties', *American Journal of Sociology*, VI/78 (May 1973), pp. 1360–80

Harrison, Robert, *Gardens: An Essay on the Human Condition* (Chicago, IL, 2008)

Hustvedt, Siri, *Living, Thinking, Looking: Essays* (New York, 2012)

Illouz, Eva, *The End of Love: A Sociology of Negative Relationships* (New York, 2019)

—, *Why Love Hurts: A Sociological Explanation* (Cambridge, 2013)

Jarman, Derek, *Derek Jarman's Garden*, photog. Howard Sooley (London, 1996)

—, *Modern Nature: The Journals of Derek Jarman, 1989–1990*, intro. Olivia Laing (London, 2018)

Kinnert, Diana, and Marc Bielefeld, *Die neue Einsamkeit: Und wie wir sie als Gesellschaft überwinden können* (Hamburg, 2021)

Klein, Melanie, 'On the Sense of Loneliness (1963)', in *Envy and Gratitude and Other Works, 1946–1963 (The Writings of Melanie Klein)* (London, 1984), pp. 300–313

van der Kolk, Bessel, *The Body Keeps the Score: Mind, Brain and Body in the Transformation of Trauma* (New York, 2015)

Kosofsky Sedgwick, Eve, *A Dialogue on Love* (Boston, MA, 1999)

—, 'Shame, Theatricality, and Queer Performativity: Henry James's *The Art of the Novel*' in David M. Halperin and Valerie Traub, *Gay Shame* (Chicago, IL, and London, 2009), pp. 49–62

Kracauer, Siegfried, *Über die Freundschaft: Essays* (Frankfurt am Main, 1978)

Krauss, Nicole, 'We're Living in a World of Walls: Here Is a Window to Escape', *New York Times* (23 October 2020)

Kristeva, Julia, *Tales of Love*, trans. Leon S. Roudiez (New York, 1987)

Laing, Olivia, *The Lonely City: Adventures in the Art of Being Alone* (Edinburgh and London, 2016)

—, *Everybody: A Book About Freedom* (London, 2021)

Lazare Mijuskovic, Ben, *Loneliness in Philosophy, Psychology and Literature* (New York, London and Amsterdam, 1979)

Lévinas, Emmanuel, *Time and the Other*, trans. Richard A. Cohen (Pittsburgh, PA, and Hamburg, 2003), 2003

Levine, Amir, and Rachel Heller, *Attached* (London, 2019)

Levy, Deborah, *Things I Don't Want to Know* (London, 2013)

—, *The Cost of Living* (London, 2018)

—, *Real Estate* (London, 2021)

Lorde, Audre, *A Burst of Light and Other Essays* (Mineola, NY, 2017)

—, *The Selected Works of Audre Lorde*, selected and with a foreword by Roxane Gay (New York, 2020)

Lyotard, Jean-François, *The Postmodern Condition: A Report on Knowledge*, trans. Geoff Bennington and Brian Massumi (Manchester, 1984)

Marquard, Odo, 'Plädoyer für die Einsamkeitsfähigkeit', in *Skepsis und Zustimmung: Philosophische Studien* (Stuttgart, 1995), pp. 110–22

Michaelis-König, Andree, and Erik Schilling, 'Poetik und Praxis der Freundschaft: Zur Einführung', *Poetik und Praxis der Freundschaft (1800–1933)* (Heidelberg, 2019), pp. 9–23

Monsour, Michael, 'The Hackneyed Notions of Adult "Same-Sex" and "Opposite-Sex" Friendships', in Mahzad Hojjat and Anne Moyer, *The Psychology of Friendship* (Oxford, 2016), pp. 59–74

Montaigne, Michel de, *Montaigne's Essays in Three Books. With Notes and Quotations. And an Account of the Author's Life.*

With a Short Character of the Author and Translator, by the Late Marquiss of Hallifax, trans. Charles Cotton (London, 1743)

Moustakas, Clark A., *Loneliness* (Englewood Cliffs, NJ, 1961)

Murthy, Vivek, *Together: The Healing Power of Human Connection in a Sometimes Lonely World* (New York, 2020)

Napoleoni, Loretta, *The Power of Knitting: Stitching Together Our Lives in a Fractured World* (New York, 2020)

Nehamas, Alexander, *On Friendship* (New York, 2016)

Nelson, Maggie, *Bluets* (London, 2017)

—, *The Red Parts: Autobiography of a Trial* (London, 2017)

Nixon, Jon, *Hannah Arendt and the Politics of Friendship* (London and New York, 2015)

Odets, Walt, *Out of the Shadows: Reimagining Gay Men's Lives* (New York, 2019)

Orbach, Susie, *Bodies* (London, 2010)

Patchett, Ann, *Truth and Beauty: A Friendship* (New York, 2004)

—, 'How Knitting Saved My Life: Twice', in *Knitting Yarns: Writers on Knitting*, ed. Ann Hood (New York and London, 2014), pp. 204–11

Philips, Adam, and Barbara Taylor, *On Kindness* (London, 2009)

Putnam, Robert, *Bowling Alone: The Collapse and Survival of American Community* (New York, 2000)

Riesman, David, *The Lonely Crowd: A Study of the Changing American Character* (Chicago, IL, 1950)

Riess, Richard, 'Freundschaft – Ferment des Lebens', in *Freundschaft* (Darmstadt, 2014)

Roach, Tom, *Friendship as a Way of Life: Foucault, AIDS, and the Politics of Shared Estrangement* (New York, 2012)

Roseneil, Sasha, 'Neue Freundschaftspraktiken: Fürsorge und Sorge um sich im Zeitalter der Individualisierung', *Mittelweg 36:*

Zeitschrift des Hamburger Instituts für Sozialforschung (*Journal of the Hamburg Institute of Social Research*), XVII/3 (June/July 2008), pp. 55–70

Rutt, Richard, *A History of Hand Knitting* (New York, 1989)

Samuel, Julia, *This Too Shall Pass: Stories of Change, Crisis and Hopeful Beginnings* (London, 2020)

Sartre, Jean-Paul, *Nausea*, trans. Robert Baldick (London, 2000)

Schinkel, Andreas, 'Das Selbst im Spiegel des Anderen: Zur Geschichte und Struktur der Freundschaft', in Dirk Villány, Matthias D. Witte and Uwe Sander, eds, *Globale Jugend und Jugendkulturen: Aufwachsen im Zeitalter der Globalisierung* (Weinheim and Munich, 2007), pp. 315–29

Schobin, Janosch, 'Sechs Farben und drei Rotationsachsen: Versuch über Verpflichtungen in Freundschaften', *Mittelweg 36: Zeitschrift des Hamburger Instituts für Sozialforschung* (*Journal of the Hamburg Institute of Social Research*), XVII/3 (June/July 2008), pp. 17–41

——, Vincenz Leuschner, Sabine Flick, Erika Alleweldt, Eric Anton Heuser and Agnes Brandt, *Freundschaft heute: Eine Einführung in die Freundschaftssoziologie* (Bielefeld, 2016), pp. 11–19

The School of Life, *On Being Nice* (London, 2017)

Selfhout Maarten, Jaap Denissen, Susan Branje and Wim Meeus, 'In the Eye of the Beholder: Perceived, Actual and Peer-Rated Similarity in Personality, Communication, and Friendship Intensity During the Acquaintanceship Process', *Journal of Personality and Social Psychology*, VI/96 (June 2009), pp. 1152–65

Solnit, Rebecca, *Wanderlust: A History of Walking* (London, 2014)

Spencer, Liz, and Ray Pahl, *Rethinking Friendship: Hidden Solidarities Today* (Princeton, NJ, and Oxford, 2006)

Stuart-Smith, Sue, *The Well-Gardened Mind: Rediscovering Nature in the Modern World* (London, 2020)

Svendsen, Lars, *A Philosophy of Loneliness* (London, 2017)

Szakolczai, Árpád, *Reflexive Historical Sociology* (London, 2000)

—, 'Permanent (Trickster) Liminality: The Reasons of the Heart and of the Mind', *Theory and Psychology*, 11/27 (April 2017), pp. 231–48

Thomassen, Bjørn, *Liminality and the Modern: Living through the In-Between* (Farnham and Burlington, VT, 2014)

Turkle, Sherry, *Alone Together: Why We Expect More from Technology and Less from Each Other* (New York, 2011)

—, *Reclaiming Conversation: The Power of Talk in a Digital Age* (New York, 2015)

Turner, Victor, *The Ritual Process: Structure and Anti-Structure* (Piscataway, NJ, 1996)

Vaillant, George E., *The Men of the Harvard Grant Study* (London, 2012)

Weil, Simone, *Amitié. L'Art de bien aimer* (Paris, 2016)

—, *Gravity and Grace*, trans. Emma Crawford and Mario von der Ruhr (London and New York, 2002)

Weiss, Douglas, *Intimacy Anorexia: Healing the Hidden Addiction in Your Marriage* (Colorado Springs, CO, 2010)

—, *Loneliness: The Experience of Emotional and Social Isolation* (Boston, MA, 1975)

Woolf, Virginia, *Street Haunting: A London Adventure* (San Francisco, CA, 1930)

Yalom, Marilyn, with Theresa Donovan Brown, *The Social Sex: A History of Female Friendship* (New York, 2015)

ACKNOWLEDGEMENTS

There are some people without whom I would not want to lead my life, this life alone. People who accompany me and are there for me whenever they can be. I am grateful to all of them. Some of them have appeared in these pages with their first names; others have remained anonymous or are present in imagined parentheses. I would like to print a list of all their names here. But I hope they know that I am talking about them and that they have a firm place in my heart.

One of these people appearing in these pages but staying anonymous is Ben Fergusson, who, in addition to being a wonderful writer, is a very talented and skilled translator and to my delight agreed to translate *Alone* into English. I cannot thank him enough – for his brilliant work, his patience with my Americanized ear battling his British diction and for his great friendship.

And finally, I'd like to especially thank Gabriele von Arnim, Sylvia Bahr, Isabel Bogdan, Theresia Enzensberger, Beatrice Fassbender, Julia Graf, Franziska Günther, Karsten Kredel, Kristof Magnusson, Lina Muzur, Marie Naumann, Maria-Christina Piwowarski, Anne Scharf, Olaf Wielk and Hanya Yanagihara. And not to forget Jacob Hochrein and Esther Mikuszies from the Goethe-Institut Nancy, and Carole Barmettler, Manuel Berger and Walter Willy Willimann from the Beau Séjour in Lucerne. We have shared many conversations about the reflections in this book, forming its foundation. They have provided me with time and emotional support in the form of writing residencies, generously shared their initial impressions of the book with me or gave me essential intellectual insight. Without them, *Alone* would not exist.